ST. JOHN'S WORT

August 1998

With Best Wishes

Norman Rosenthal

Also by Norman Rosenthal, M.D.

Winter Blues

ST. JOHN'S WORT

WORT

The Herbal Way to Feeling Good

NORMAN ROSENTHAL, M.D.

HarperCollins*Publishers*

HarperCollins books may be purchased for educational, business, or sales promotional use. For information please write: Special Markets Department, HarperCollins Publishers, Inc., 10 East 53rd Street, New York, NY 10022.

FIRST EDITION

Designed by Nancy Singer Olaguera

Library of Congress Cataloging-in-Publication Data

Rosenthal, Norman, M.D.
    St. John's wort : the herbal way to feeling good / Norman Rosenthal, M.D.
      p.   cm.
    Includes bibliographical reference and index.
    ISBN 0-06-018382-9
    1. Depression, Mental—Alternative treatment. 2. Hypericum perforatum—Therapeutic use. I. Title.
    RC537.R6386 1998
    616.85'2706—dc21   98-21686

98 99 00 01 02 v/RRD 10 9 8 7 6 5 4 3 2 1

For Jean

It is hard to describe how great and important the character [of St. John's wort] is and how great it may be in the future.

—PARACELSUS, 1493–1541,
COLLECTED WRITINGS

In various patients I have found these effects and, without overstating the herb's benefits, I effected cures which you achieve neither with all the rest of your Apothecary nor with the best prescriptions made out of gold, silver, coral, pearls, stone or jewels (even those that have been found to be useful and wonderful in the treatment of other illnesses).

—ANGELO SALA, 1576–1637, *ESSENTIARUM VEGETABILIUM ANATOME*

After six years of solid depression, of feeling crippled and at the edge of a cliff, ready to jump . . . all my ailments have subsided. I no longer feel any need for a medical professional. My faith has been restored. It's a miracle.

—ST. JOHN'S WORT USER, 1997

CONTENTS

Contents

ACKNOWLEDGMENTS

Thanks and acknowledgment are due to the many people who helped in various stages of the preparation of this book. Jean Carper gave me the idea to write it and helped each step of the way. Drs. Siegfried Kasper, Hans-Peter Volz, David Wheatley, and Franz Mueller-Spähn were kind enough to share their clinical experience with me, and Dr. Walter Müller shared his pharmacological expertise. Dr. Alexander Neumeister translated German texts and personally conducted interviews in Germany on my behalf. Drs. Thomas Wehr and Jeremy Waletzky gave generously of their ideas and referred patients to me. Dr. Alice Phillips provided helpful suggestions. Dr. Kay Redfield Jamison was an inspiration, as always. Dr. Judith Rapoport, Jerolyn Ross, and Helen Wall carefully read and edited the manuscript. Joshua Rosenthal, Stacey Chok, and Joanne Milne helped as research assistants. Thanks to my editors at HarperCollins, Vice President and Associate Publisher Gladys Justin Carr and Elissa Altman; and to my agent, Raphael Sagalyn. My wife, Dr. Leora Rosen, gave invaluable support and suggestions. And, finally, thanks to the many patients who shared their experiences with the herbal antidepressant, without whose anonymous contribution this book would not have been possible.

INTRODUCTION

If you have suffered from depression, you know the pain and frustration of trying to escape from its black depths. Even if you just have occasional mild attacks of the blues, for example, premenstrually or during the dark days of winter, you can appreciate the changes in brain chemistry that bring on the distressing down moods. Of course, drugs to change that brain chemistry are establishment medicine's main way of treating depression.

But now, a new and very exciting drug—not from the major pharmaceutical companies but from nature's own pharmacy, and widely used and researched in Europe—is beginning to make waves in the United States. It is St. John's wort, or hypericum. And it promises to be as big here in the United States as it is in Europe. It is currently available over the counter, and a major multicenter research trial, funded by the National Institute of Mental Health, is soon to be started. But it will be years before the results of this study will be available as a guide for those who might stand to benefit from the herb. In the meantime, most U.S. psychiatrists are unaccustomed to the use of this novel antidepressant and there is a tremendous need for detailed information about the herb and its uses. In this book, my goal is to provide up-to-date information on what is currently known about St. John's wort and how best to use it, based on my review of all the available literature, both ancient and modern, extensive interviews with European colleagues, direct surveys of many who have used St. John's wort without medical supervision, and my own clinical experience.

If studies in the United States confirm European research findings, and the U.S. public has access to good information about the herbal remedy, St. John's wort may emerge as one of the most popular, effective, and safe of antidepressants. And there's no reason to think that St. John's wort will not work on Americans fully as well as on Europeans. In Germany, St.

John's wort is the number one antidepressant prescribed by physicians, far outselling Prozac by more than ten times over. Every year, German doctors write 3 million prescriptions for St. John's wort as compared with 240,000 prescriptions for Prozac. This widespread usage is all the more remarkable considering that the herb has become widely prescribed in Germany just in the past decade. In this book, I will provide you with insights into some of the unique features of this herbal antidepressant that explain its popularity in Europe and its growing appeal here in the United States as well.

Depression can be an extremely serious condition and, in some cases, may be fatal. It is estimated to affect 17.6 million people in the United States and to cost the country 43 billion dollars each year. Any new advance that offers to lessen the burden of this illness, both for those who suffer from it and for society at large, is a welcome development. At the same time, it is important for an individual who may be suffering from the condition to recognize it and seek proper help when this is necessary. I hope to provide those who might be suffering from depression with guidance as to when it is imperative to bring a qualified professional into the picture.

In addition, I will describe the potential value of St. John's wort in many types of situations for which systematic research is not as yet available, but where an accumulation of individual anecdotes suggests promising new clinical uses for the herb. These include the stresses of everyday life, winter depression, also known as seasonal affective disorder (SAD), depression in the elderly, and a host of other conditions such as panic disorder, extreme shyness or social phobia, insomnia, and compulsive hair pulling.

What Is Unique About St. John's Wort?

There are several unique features of St. John's wort.

- St. John's wort is the product of nature's own pharmacy rather than the result of pharmaceutical developments.

- Unlike some untested herbal remedies, St. John's wort really does appear to work.

- It has an unusually mild and acceptable side-effect profile.

- It appears to have a unique pharmacological action.

- It is available over the counter, unlike all other antidepressants, which require a doctor's prescription.

- It has an amazing history and mythology extending back almost two thousand years.

So, paradoxically, the latest antidepressant is also the first effective medicine ever to have been used in the pharmacological treatment of depression. Each of these unique qualities is worth considering.

The Appeal of Natural Treatments

There is tremendous interest in this country in alternative medicine, including the healing powers of herbs, and with good reason. Many conventional medicines originally came from herbs. For example, the heart-boosting drug digitalis was originally extracted from the leaves of the foxglove plant, and the antidiarrheal medicine atropine from the root of the deadly nightshade plant. More recently, we have seen the discovery of the amazing anticancer drug tamoxifen, derived from the bark of the Pacific yew tree. So it should not come as a complete surprise that the vast plant kingdom, with its approximately 8 million distinct species, should yield an effective antidepressant as well.

For centuries herbalists and medicine men from many different cultures have attributed healing powers to a multitude of herbs. Recognizing the need to systematize this wisdom and subject it to some of the scrutiny and rigors of modern science, the former German Federal Health Agency appointed a group of scientists and medical experts to develop an inventory of herbs for which there was reasonable evidence of some medicinal efficacy. That led to Commission E, which published a report produced in Germany in the mid-1980s stating that approximately three hundred herbs appeared to be effective in the treatment of a variety of conditions. German scientists concluded that one of the most promising of these was St. John's wort, and in the past five to ten years, many scientific studies have been devoted to its beneficial effects in the treatment of depression.

Scientific Evidence That St. John's Wort Works

To date there have been over two dozen studies of the efficacy of St. John's wort as an antidepressant, all of them done in Europe. I will discuss them later in the book. The simple conclusion to be drawn from these studies is that it is an effective antidepressant with a very favorable side-effect profile. Of course, there are questions that remain to be answered by proper scientific studies. How does St. John's wort compare in efficacy and side effects with the most widely used antidepressants, Prozac and Zoloft? Can the herbal antidepressant be combined with other antidepressants to take advantage of their different qualities? What is the best way to switch from a conventional antidepressant to St. John's wort, and should you consider switching at all? Even though science has not yet provided satisfactory answers to these questions, they are of compelling clinical interest and we need to provide the best answers possible based on the knowledge available to us at this time. I address all these questions in the pages of this book.

St. John's Wort May Have a Unique Mode of Pharmacological Action

The most popular antidepressants currently on the market, including Prozac and Zoloft, act almost exclusively on the neurotransmitter (nerve chemical messenger) serotonin. Available evidence suggests that St. John's wort acts not only on serotonin, but on two other key neurotransmitters as well. This broader spectrum of actions may carry with it certain advantages that explain why St. John's wort has proven to be uniquely helpful for certain individuals.

It Is the Only Antidepressant Available Over the Counter

St. John's wort is now widely available to the U.S. public in exactly the same formulation and with the same level of purity as the German version of the compound. As a botanical treatment, it falls under government regulations that permit it to be distributed over the counter, without a physician's prescription. This presents a novel opportunity for the estimated 17 million Americans who suffer from depression, many of whom will not find their way to a physician or be treated appropriately. For the first time, the U.S. public can identify and treat their own depressions with an effective antidepressant. It is as though such conventional antidepressants as Prozac or Zoloft were suddenly made directly available to the general public. But along with the opportunity comes a hazard that must be acknowledged if we are to make the most of this novel development. Self-treatment of depression can be a risky business. It is therefore critical to recognize at what points it really is imperative to seek medical attention.

For the depressed person who would previously not have sought medical help, perhaps for financial reasons or out of feelings of shame or the fear of stigma, St. John's wort might well be a boon. On the other hand, a seriously depressed person who really needs the wisdom, support, and guidance of a skilled psychiatrist may set out to self-medicate unsuccessfully, delay recovery, and in the process suffer all manner of setbacks.

In the best of all possible worlds, everyone would have access to a first-rate psychiatrist, someone who would be available, affordable, empathic, and knowledgeable, someone who would be there to listen to your sorrows, advise you judiciously, and help steer you through all the difficulties that depression presents. Unlike Candide, Voltaire's irrepressibly optimistic hero, most of us know that we do not live in the best of all possible worlds. Some people don't have the money to get the help they need, and sometimes the help they get is not first-rate. My hope is that this book will provide the information necessary both to enable the reader to evaluate whether a self-help approach to the treatment of depression makes sense, and to judge when and how to involve a professional in the treatment plan. Sometimes the inclusion of a professional is critical; at other times, perhaps, optional.

Whether or not you choose to seek out the help of a professional, I hope you find the information in this book to be useful. An open-minded therapist will appreciate a knowledgeable client. I know that I always do and often paraphrase for my patients the advertising slogan of a large discount clothing store—that an educated consumer is my best customer.

One problem with depression is that it can make you feel helpless and powerless. Obtaining knowledge about how you can fight depression is one way of regaining a sense of mastery. As you take each successive step toward combating it, you will begin to turn the problem around and feel increasingly better, closer and closer to recovery. One critical step toward doing that is straightening out the chemical problem that is at the basis of depression. St. John's wort offers a new way of doing just that. As a psychiatrist who has treated hundreds of depressed patients over the years, I have come to appreciate that good treatment of depression is a multifaceted enterprise. It is always useful to combine medical treatments of depression with nonpharmacological approaches, and I devote a chapter to the discussion of promoting an antidepressant lifestyle. I believe that the use of St. John's wort—or any antidepressant— can be greatly augmented by adding other self-care strategies to the treatment regimen.

Finally, it is important to recognize that you may not be able to treat your own depression effectively, even with St. John's wort and the most diligent use of all available self-help strategies. If that should happen, it really is critical to get professional help. Depression is a costly and hazardous condition. In the tradition of knowing your adversary, it is worth treating it with respect and mustering all available weaponry against it.

This book is divided into three parts. In the first, I tell the stories of various people whose lives have been enhanced by the herbal remedy and illustrate the many ways in which St. John's wort can help overcome depression and other conditions. I also discuss the latest research on the herb and explain how we think it works. In the second part, I help the reader develop a game plan for identifying the presence of depression and using St. John's wort as a way of treating the condition; I also show how the herb can be incorporated into an overall antidepressant lifestyle. In addition, I answer some of the questions that I have been asked most frequently about the herb and its uses. Finally, in part 3, I chronicle the fascinating history of the herb, from the observations of ancient authorities to modern times. In addition, I discuss the political and economic implications of the growing use of the herbal antidepressant.

IMPORTANT NOTE

This book is intended as a resource to educate the reader about St. John's wort and how to use the herbal remedy in an informed and effective way to overcome depression and enhance the quality of life. This book is not intended as a substitute for medical care. Depression can be a serious condition for which a good doctor or therapist is invaluable and sometimes indispensable. The reader is advised to consult his or her medical or health professional in matters relating to his or her health and particularly regarding any symptoms that may require medical attention.

This book is based on the personal experiences, research, and observations of the author. Although every effort has been made to ensure that drug selections and dosages match current recommendations and practices, because of ongoing research and other factors, the reader is cautioned to check with a health professional about specific recommendations. Anyone with a known disease or serious health condition or who is taking prescription medications should especially seek professional medical advice before taking the natural remedy described in this book. There could be interactions between the natural remedy and other drugs. Also, it should be noted that all dosages discussed in this book apply to adults, not children, unless otherwise stated.

All active remedies, whether natural or synthetic, can produce adverse effects, both short- and long-term. If you notice any such adverse affects from the use of this remedy, you should report them to your doctor without delay. The author and publisher expressly disclaim responsibility for any adverse effects arising from the use or application of the information contained in this book.

Part I

ST. JOHN'S WORT AT WORK

Success Stories

1

IT REALLY WORKS

Although a common maxim holds that "seeing is believing," the statement is actually not always true. Seeing can be quite deceptive, as anyone knows who has witnessed the tricks of a competent magician. Conversely, we believe many things that we do not actually see; for example, that the earth revolves around the sun. But in some ways, the maxim carries the weight of truth. Those things that we cannot see are hard to believe, which is one reason why they gave poor Galileo such a hard time when he maintained that the sun and not the earth was the center of the solar system. Similarly, controlled treatment studies can appear quite unconvincing if one doesn't believe in the treatment and the studies are performed by someone with ideas that differ from yours. I encountered this phenomenon after conducting numerous light-treatment studies in patients with seasonal affective disorder (SAD), or winter depression. The studies from my group at the National Institute of Mental Health, as well as those of numerous colleagues, told a clear story. Light therapy worked. Yet many psychiatrists who had never treated a single patient with light therapy remained skeptical. But the successful treatment of a single patient with this modality was in certain instances more persuasive than all the published data on the topic. So, after studying SAD for several years and treating many hundreds of patients with light therapy, I was amused when an old colleague approached me at a meeting and said to me with an air of discovery, "You know that light therapy that you have been talking about all this time? I treated a patient with it and the darn thing works."

In truth, though, it is wonderful to discover a phenomenon

for oneself even if it has been described a thousand times before. And so it was for me with the use of St. John's wort in depression. I had read about controlled studies performed in Europe and had actually seen some of the data. Yet it was only when I saw some of my own patients benefit from the herbal remedy that I felt the excitement that might be expected to greet the arrival of a novel form of treatment for an old and nasty adversary—depression.

Fired by a Pharmacist's Assistant

"This letter is to cancel my appointment," wrote Malcolm*, who worked as an assistant to a pharmacist. "I suppose I could come in and 'show myself to the priest' . . . but I had only mild to moderate depressions, not leprosy. . . . I have never been a danger to myself or others, only a danger to my checkbook. And in the interests of protecting my checking account, I would like to cancel further appointments.

"I am relatively happy with my current 'prescription' of St. John's wort. It is working as well as, or better than, any of the antidepressants I have tried so far. So I'll keep with it for now, and see how well it does as the days get longer. If I feel the need to try more prescriptions, I will feel free to call."

Well, I have always encouraged my patients to express themselves freely to me and apparently Malcolm had taken me at my word. But his letter captured my attention more for its substance than its style. Malcolm's depression had been very difficult to treat. It was not that his symptoms were so severe. He was correct in describing them as mild to moderate and he had never felt suicidal, but it was long-standing and seemed to sap his life of all joy. His energy level was very low and he withdrew from others in order to conserve his meager energy reserves for his job. His only pleasure came from buying things, such as compact discs. "Music seemed to fill my emptiness," he

---

*The names of all patients used throughout this book are pseudonyms.

said. Two women he had dated over the previous ten years had remarked that his main problem was that he wasn't happy, though he was barely aware of this unhappiness himself.

I had treated Malcolm's symptoms with a comprehensive list of antidepressant medications, trying each one diligently for the right amount of time, calibrating dosages, using novel and unusual combinations, and integrating the medications with all sorts of health-enhancing recommendations. While these interventions were quite helpful, we were always brought up short by side effects, especially problems with his sinuses, dryness of the mouth, and feelings of spaciness. Of all the medications we had used, Zoloft seemed best, but he still felt unhappy and "out of touch" emotionally. He decided to stop Zoloft after finding out about St. John's wort on the World Wide Web and concluded that he had enough information on which to base an intelligent decision.

Malcolm followed his earlier communication to me with a second letter to reassure me that "I was in no way displeased with your 'psychiatric care' (I guess the term is)" and to report on "my current herbal concoction." He was now on hypericum, 900 milligrams (mg) per day, which appeared both to reduce his anxiety and to energize him. He was "more positive and upbeat, more apt to say goofy things instead of sitting around and being quiet." He was amazed to find himself more outgoing and confident, even among strangers. He felt a qualitative difference between the effects of Zoloft and those of St. John's wort. While the Zoloft had helped his mood, it had not allowed him to communicate that improved mood to others and to engage with them as freely as was now possible.

Over the next six months, while taking St. John's wort, Malcolm made certain changes in his life. He made sure to get enough sleep, which helped his energy level, and kept his time of waking constant even on weekend days, which he believed had a marked stabilizing effect on his mood. He left the pharmacy, where he had felt isolated, and took up a job in a home for mentally retarded adults, where he had more daily contact with people. He involved himself in religious activities, which added a spiritual dimension to his life. Finally, he plucked up the courage to approach a young lady whom he had met at church and whom he is now dating.

My experience with Malcolm was my first direct encounter with the new herbal antidepressant and to say that I was amazed would be an understatement. After treating him with so many potent antidepressants, both individually and in combination, and observing his responses to them, I discounted a placebo explanation for his improvement. In his case, I was convinced that the herb had exerted a specific antidepressant effect. Even so, his story reminded me once again of how important it is to add healthy activities to any antidepressant intervention, but I again realized how little these activities may help unless the disturbance in brain chemistry has been turned around.

It is possible that the tendency of St. John's wort to make Malcolm more outgoing might have been related to its effects on the neurotransmitter dopamine, which is important in regulating social behavior in animals. We will see this beneficial effect of St. John's wort in some of the other people profiled in this book. The mood-enhancing effects that Malcolm experienced on both Zoloft and St. John's wort might have been related to the effects of both of these substances on another neurotransmitter, serotonin. The role of these neurotransmitters and the effects of St. John's wort on them are discussed further in chapter 4.

The lessons I learned from Malcolm encouraged me to try St. John's wort in my practice. The first patient I treated was Adele, whose story I describe below.

Adele: Lessons from an Anxious Educator

Adele is a woman of approximately fifty whom I have treated for the past eight years. Although extremely intelligent, she had experienced learning difficulties since childhood, which she mastered sufficiently to complete college and graduate school successfully and become an educator herself, teaching others how to teach. Despite the many good things in her life—a loving husband, children of whom she is proud, good looks, and physical health—Adele has suffered long stretches of time during which she has felt tired, tearful, and, above all, anxious. During these times she would lose interest and initiative, have trouble sleeping, be unable to concentrate on her work, and devalue herself.

These episodes of depression and anxiety would come and go over the years, sometimes, apparently, with the seasons, sometimes in response to stress, and sometimes for no good discernible reason at all. And over the years I had treated Adele with a series of antidepressants, all of which had created problems that, sooner or later, were deal-breakers and she would elect to discontinue the medications rather than suffer the side effects. Prozac caused her to itch unbearably. Wellbutrin made her edgy and irritable. Zoloft stripped her of her sex drive and ability to have orgasms. Light therapy in winter was of some help but not sufficient in itself. Psychotherapy helped her deal with some of her life issues, many of which were the result of childhood sorrows and traumas, but didn't resolve the symptoms of her underlying depression—fatigue to the point of exhaustion, sadness, and, in the background, all-encompassing anxiety.

After my experience with Malcolm's self-treatment, I began to take the European literature on St. John's wort more seriously. I was eager for Adele to try the herb, as her depressive symptoms seemed to fit the profile of those who had most frequently benefited from the drug. I gave her some samples of Jarsin, the type of St. John's wort used in most of the European research literature and now available in the United States under the brand name of Kira, with instructions based on the advice of my German colleagues. Neither of us could have hoped for a happier outcome. Within weeks of starting St. John's wort, 300 mg twice a day, Adele began to feel more confident, content, and optimistic. Her anxiety disappeared and, best of all, she experienced no side effects. The return of sexual feelings and the ability to express and enjoy them were extremely welcome developments. Although her job had been a long-standing source of conflict for her, suddenly she felt that it offered her new opportunities that she had not previously appreciated. As far as Adele is concerned, St. John's wort has opened up a whole new world of possibilities for someone who has fought a long and painful battle with depression and anxiety.

The stories of Malcolm and Adele were my introduction to the surprisingly potent effects of St. John's wort, but they were just the beginning of my positive experiences with the herbal antidepressant. The chapters that follow describe some of the many people with a variety of problems who have benefited from St. John's wort, as well as specific guidance as to how you might benefit from it too.

2

ST. JOHN'S WORT IN EVERYDAY LIFE

Information about the effects of St. John's wort on people entering research protocols and those seeking help from psychiatrists gives us only a very partial picture about how the herbal remedy is being used. The large majority of people who have turned to the herb would probably never qualify for a research protocol nor see fit to consult a psychiatrist. How is St. John's wort being used by the general public, and how is it working for the problems of everyday life? Those are questions that I wanted to answer. In order to do so, I surveyed the public directly by means of a questionnaire distributed in health food stores and pharmacies both in the United States and in Germany and posted on certain Internet news groups. Many people responded and, based on their answers, it is apparent that people are using St. John's wort—and finding it to be helpful—for such diverse types of discomfort as work stress, mild cases of the blues, insomnia, premenstrual syndrome, and extreme shyness. Reluctant to seek medical help for these ailments, many are helping themselves with this herbal remedy. Here are some of their stories.

Combating Work Stress with St. John's Wort

From the dark realms of cyberspace, a nineteen-year-old girl who calls herself Dream writes to me as follows:

> I began taking St. John's wort, 600–900 mg per day, for depression—severe mood swings, excessive anger, guilt, feelings of worthlessness and irritability. It helped me function at work. My job requires good customer rela-

tions, and I was too easily irritated and pissed off. On St. John's wort I could smile and interact just fine. It caused me a problem only once when I took it on an empty stomach and suffered severe stomach cramps for the rest of the day. I've stopped taking St. John's wort because I feel better now. I was extremely grateful for it because it enabled me to function at work and subsequently keep my job (I recently got promoted too). I can't afford a doctor or any expensive medications. I only wish St. John's wort worked as well for everyone else as it did for me.

Work stress is a common source of frustration in modern times. Perhaps it always has been. But nowadays, corporate downsizing is making many workers increasingly insecure about their jobs. International competition has led to companies trying to get as much from their workers as possible for as little as possible. People shoved into *Dilbert*-type work cubicles feel unappreciated and depersonalized. Chronic stress results in both physical and behavioral changes. Physically, there may be evidence of increased tension, and blood pressure and pulse rate may rise. More stress hormones, such as cortisol, are produced by the adrenal gland, which can reduce appetite and disrupt sleep. After time, an individual can feel burned out and, like the woman in the above anecdote, can become irritable in ways that can get her into trouble with her supervisor. If stress continues for long enough, it can turn into clinical depression, and a person would do well to head off such a development at the pass. There are, of course, many things one can do to reduce stress and avoid depression, as outlined in chapter 11. But one easy solution, which should certainly be considered, is the use of St. John's wort. As in Dream's experience, the need for the herb may be temporary, to tide a person over a particularly stressful time, but the benefits may be permanent. For example, in Dream's case, she was promoted, perhaps as a result of the improved mood and better control of her temper while on the herbal remedy.

Unemployment

Although work-related problems are stressful, getting fired, laid off, downsized, or whatever it is called nowadays can be even more so. For example, a forty-eight-year-old man from Germany who has treated himself with St. John's wort for the past year writes, "I lost my job a year ago. I was finished with the world. Now, after a month in a new job, I am fine. With all the problems I was having, I could no longer see light at the end of the tunnel. Now everything is normal again." There are all sorts of adjustments that need to be made following a job loss and specific actions that need to be taken to determine how best to find new employment or get on with one's career. But putting your brain chemicals in order may be a first step in developing the best mind-set to enable you to make these changes; for this person from Germany, St. John's wort appears to have done just that.

Loss and Bereavement

Another source of chronic stress is the aftermath of losing a loved one. Grieving is an extremely painful process but probably a valuable and necessary one. Nevertheless, in some people the degree of suffering is so great that some form of medication may be warranted. In one recent study of widows and widowers, researchers found that almost one in four of the bereaved individuals had enough symptoms to be given the diagnosis of full-blown clinical depression. The decision as to whether to alleviate such painful symptoms is obviously a personal one. For many people, the idea of a natural substance, an herbal antidepressant that they can buy and administer themselves, may prove to be appealing. A forty-five-year-old woman from Germany described how she had taken St. John's wort three times a day to deal with her feelings of grief following the death of her husband six months before. She felt that St. John's wort helped her enormously; now she is more at peace with herself and can sleep properly again.

Illness in a Loved One

The chronic illness of a close relative or friend and the unremitting care and attention it may require is another stress that can wear down those who love the ailing person. For example, a sixty-four-year-old German woman felt very stressed as a result of her husband's depression. Taking St. John's wort in the usual dosage of 300 mg three times a day has helped her enormously without causing any side effects. Now she feels better and can sleep again.

Although there are no research studies on the use of St. John's wort for the treatment of stress, it is commonplace to recommend conventional antidepressants for such off-prescription uses, often to very good effect. Already there are thousands of people using St. John's wort for chronic stress. I predict that its use in this regard will greatly increase over the coming decade.

Chasing Away the Blues: The Common and Distressing Problem of Subsyndromal Depression

While depression is in itself a common condition for many people—according to one estimate, it affects about one in ten people in any given year—many others are affected by depressive symptoms to a degree that would not qualify them for the more serious diagnosis. According to Dr. Lewis Judd, former director of the National Institute of Mental Health, and colleagues, approximately one in five people interviewed in a 1994 study reported having suffered from one or more depressive symptoms in the preceding month. The most common of these symptoms are shown in the following table, together with their frequency in the month before the interview.

trouble falling asleep, staying asleep, waking early	34 percent
feeling tired all the time	23 percent

thought a lot about death	23 percent
two weeks sad, blue, or depressed	12 percent
increased appetite, gained as much as two pounds a week	9.5 percent
interest in sex less than usual	9.5 percent
a lot more trouble concentrating	9 percent
sleeping too much	8 percent

If you think about the implications of these figures for a moment, they really are quite staggering. Huge numbers of people are suffering from very distressing problems of mood, behavior, and bodily functions of the type that are associated with depression. Nor are these symptoms benign in terms of their impact on a person's functioning. Judd and colleagues found that people with subsyndromal depression reported more difficulties in their work and social relationships and that significantly more people with these symptoms had been on disability. Given the reluctance that people have to seek medical attention even for full-blown cases of depression, and the poor medical care they frequently receive once they make such a decision, it seems unlikely that a high percentage of people with subsyndromal depression will be properly treated through conventional medical channels. Such people are therefore excellent candidates for self-treatment with St. John's wort, and there is no reason to believe that it will not prove to be helpful for many of them, given its excellent track record in more severely depressed patients.

St. John's Wort and Insomnia

As I have noted, insomnia is one of the most commonly reported disturbances in behavior. As the above table indicates, as many as one in three people report that in the previous month they have had some problem related to their sleep patterns. Many people, especially from Germany, wrote to tell me that they had taken St. John's wort, to good effect, to treat their insomnia. For example, a fifty-two-year-old woman began to take St. John's wort "because I was not sleeping when it was possible to do so." Since starting St. John's wort "I don't stay awake if I wake up during the night unless there is an emergency. It also reinforces my positive outlook during the day."

It is important to remember that sleep difficulties are a cardinal symptom of depression. These difficulties may take the form of having trouble falling asleep, tossing and turning or sleeping fitfully during the night, or awakening too early in the morning. So distressing are such symptoms that they may overwhelm the clinical picture and the depressed person may diagnose the condition as insomnia.

All types of antidepressants may be helpful in reversing insomnia when it is part of the overall picture of depression. St. John's wort is no exception in this regard. People with insomnia might benefit from reading over the symptoms of depression, as outlined in chapter 8, to determine whether they are suffering from other symptoms of depression as well. If they are, then the herbal remedy is more likely to help resolve their sleep difficulties.

A fifty-six-year-old woman writes to tell me how her sleep difficulties, which were the most troublesome symptoms of her depression, were helped by St. John's wort. "I can sleep again!" she exclaims. "Getting rest at night has helped everything else; gloom has lifted and I am in good spirits, energetic and positive. I feel a heavy weight off me. Immediately (the first night) I began to have dreams. I used to dream lots until about five to six years ago when menopause kicked in. I did not dream as usual, if at all. I really hadn't thought about it until I took St. John's wort and began to dream again. Maybe the increased dreams are related to feeling better also."

If there are no other symptoms of depression, however, the insomnia may well be due to some other condition. It is worth paying a visit to the doctor to have the problem checked out as some causes of insomnia are potentially dangerous and eminently treatable. One such cause is sleep apnea, a condition in which people stop breathing for brief spells frequently during the night, which wakes them up repeatedly. This leaves people drowsy and hungover during the day, thus putting them at risk when driving or operating machinery. The resulting lack of oxygen to the tissues can also be medically harmful. Sleep apnea is unlikely to respond to St. John's wort, but can readily be treated by other means, such as a special machine that pumps air into the lungs when a person stops breathing.

Simple but important factors worth considering in identifying possible causes of insomnia include commonly used drugs such as caffeine, nicotine, and alcohol. Often cutting down the number of cups of coffee or tea or caffeinated sodas, particularly in the later part of the day, can work wonders in bringing insomnia under control. Some people may not realize that nicotine is a stimulant and that smoking in the later part of the evening may be preventing them from falling asleep. And even though alcohol has immediate sedative properties, its effects wear off after a few hours. Too much alcohol at night may appear to promote sleep but may actually disrupt it when blood alcohol levels begin to fall. Removing these drugs from the later part of the day or, at times, altogether can be very helpful in promoting restful sleep. In addition, sleep experts emphasize the importance of what they call sleep hygiene—a quiet, peaceful bedroom with dim lights and low noise levels. They recommend keeping arguments and conflicts out of the bedroom late at night and engaging in peaceful rituals to wind oneself down before bedtime. If such simple remedies don't help overcome sleep difficulties in the absence of depressive symptoms, it is worth seeking out the help of an appropriate physician. If insomnia is part of a depression, however, it may resolve when treated with St. John's wort or an antidepressant.

Taking the Edge off PMS

It is estimated that approximately 5 percent of women of childbearing age have serious mood difficulties during the several days before their periods. Millions more suffer to a lesser degree. Is it possible that St. John's wort might help many of these women feel good all month long? According to some of the responses to my survey, the answer appears to be yes.

One young woman wrote to tell me that she had started the herbal remedy specifically for mood difficulties related to her periods. After six months of treatment with 600 mg of St. John's wort per day, she now regards her moods as stable, though not perfect. Although she still feels bad at times, she has a sense of being in control of her emotions, and that makes all the difference. According to her, St. John's wort has helped "an incredible amount," without any side effects whatsoever. A woman colleague similarly informed me that St. John's wort "took the bottoms off my PMS symptoms."

Given the success of St. John's wort as an antidepressant, these findings of beneficial effects on PMS should come as no surprise, since other antidepressants have also proved to be helpful in controlling the monthly symptoms of this disorder. Despite the potential payoff of continuous antidepressant usage on PMS, many of my patients with this condition understandably balk at taking medications and suffering their side effects all month long to forestall symptoms that persist for only a small (though very unpleasant) portion of the month. Since St. John's wort is very easily tolerated by most people, it may prove to be a boon for such individuals, who might view it as an innocuous herbal supplement rather than a potent medication with unpleasant side effects.

Fear of Humiliation: St. John's Wort and Social Phobia

Social phobia, one of the most common hidden causes of distress and anxiety in everyday life, is estimated to affect approximately one in eight U.S. adults. People with this problem have a persistent and powerful fear of being scrutinized, evaluated, or judged by others. As you can imagine, this condition results in considerable impairment of functioning, as it prevents people from asserting themselves in their work situations and making social overtures. Although people with this difficulty may simply appear shy to outsiders, they actually spend a great deal of time worrying about being embarrassed and engage in painful fantasies of being ridiculed or humiliated.

According to Dr. Michael Liebowitz of Columbia University, a pioneering researcher in the field of social phobia, there are several lines of evidence suggesting that brain pathways involving the neurotransmitter dopamine are disturbed in social phobia. To a somewhat lesser extent, pathways involving serotonin also seem to be involved in this condition. Studies indicate that antidepressants may be of some value in the treatment of social phobia. Because St. John's wort has been shown to influence both dopamine and serotonin transmission, as explained in chapter 4, there is reason to predict that the herbal remedy might be of some benefit in social phobia. As several of the stories in this book will indicate, after starting the herbal remedy, people report becoming more outgoing and less shy, more willing to risk taking the initiative in a social or work situation.

Currently, social phobia is a greatly undertreated problem, in part because it is not recognized by clinicians but perhaps also because the very symptoms of the condition—fear of being judged and humiliated—may prevent people from bringing their problem to the attention of a professional. For these people, an herbal remedy that can be purchased over the counter is likely to be enormously appealing. Although formal studies of this use of the herb for social phobia are needed, early evidence suggests that if you are painfully shy or afraid of making a social overture or asserting yourself, St. John's wort may really be worth a try.

As we can see, there are many possible roles for St. John's wort in everyday life—for stress, low energy, down feelings, insomnia, premenstrual symptoms, and painful shyness. Small wonder that the ancients thought the herb capable of miracles and attributed magical powers to it. But though helpful for relatively minor conditions, St. John's wort can also be surprisingly powerful for severe depression as well, as illustrated by the more serious cases in the next chapter.

3

THE PROZAC OF HERBS

Just as St. John's wort is versatile in its capacity to alleviate relatively minor psychological ailments, so it appears to be effective for people suffering from a broad spectrum of more severe psychiatric disorders. In this chapter I relate the stories of a few of these people, who were either referred to me by colleagues or who answered my questionnaire.

For the benefit of skeptics, perhaps it is fitting that our first story should be that of a man who was successfully treated for his depression without his knowledge. Although I am not in favor of medicating people on the sly nor wish to encourage dissatisfied spouses to engage in duplicitous behavior, I could not resist including a story that is so instructive and has such a happy ending.

Meet Sam, a depressed lawyer; Sylvia, his concerned wife; and her close friend Louise, a woman of great resourcefulness, who happens to be a patient of mine.

St. John's Wort in the Breakfast Vitamins: A Single Blind Study

Louise, a professional woman who has been in treatment with me for several years, has, in the course of this time, become knowledgeable about the administration and regulation of antidepressant medications and, as a consequence, is much sought after by friends and family members for her opinions in this regard even though she has no formal medical training. Accordingly, she was consulted by her friend Sylvia in connection with Sylvia's husband's difficulties. Sylvia believed that

Sam, her husband, was suffering from depression because he seemed "down in the dumps, sat in front of the television till late at night, and self-medicated with junk food—anything he could eat without cooking; anything that came in a box, such as our baby's crackers and pretzels." In addition, he was having a hard time getting to sleep at night, was staying up till the early hours of the morning, and was isolating himself. She was worried because he had previously been a very optimistic person, believing the world to be essentially a good place, full of opportunities, before a series of business reversals had set off these changes in him. She knew that several members on both sides of his family had suffered from depression. When he barricaded himself in the bedroom one night, a highly unusual thing for him to do, Sylvia had reached her limit. It was time to consult Louise.

The idea of suggesting that Sam go to a psychiatrist was completely impractical to Sylvia. "He didn't think there was anything wrong with him," she explained. "He would never have gone and wouldn't have considered taking Prozac or any other antidepressant." How might she handle such a refractory patient, she asked Louise in one of their regular phone calls. Based on her readings about depression, Louise suggested that Sam try St. John's wort.

The idea was immediately appealing to Sylvia, but certain logistical problems presented themselves. First, she was unable to get her hands on St. John's wort in the small town where they lived and, second, she knew Sam to be highly suggestible and she wanted to make sure that the herb was really working and that she was not instead dealing with some half-baked placebo effect. Louise told her that the first problem could be easily solved, as she would send Sylvia the right type of St. John's wort. As to the placebo effect, Louise inquired about Sam's daily activities and on discovering that he was in the habit of taking vitamins every morning with breakfast, suggested that Sylvia simply inform Sam that the St. John's wort tablets were additional vitamins and add them to the mix. Sylvia approved of the plan. She knew that Sam was generally distracted by work-related matters at breakfast time and, not being by nature a suspicious person, would readily take whatever tablets Sylvia gave him. "He's lucky I like him," she observed, adding, "I'm a suspicious person; you could never get away with giving me extra pills." Nevertheless, she could not push her luck too far and ask him to take vitamins in the evening, which would have constituted a major change in his daily activities and would have elicited suspicion even in a highly trusting husband. In addition, as she noted, "I have no control over his lunch." So even though St. John's wort is supposed to be administered three times a day, Sylvia decided he would have to take all three tablets at breakfast. She knew that the herbal remedy was best taken with food and reckoned that "if he got sick, it would be immediate and I would know what it was." She was pleased to see that he tolerated the new pills just fine.

After about five to six weeks, Sylvia noticed a remarkable improvement in Sam's mood and demeanor, which she characterized as "happy but not manic." He became "more balanced, grounded, present and alive, better than he has been in years." He stopped watching as much television, picked up his old musical interests again, playing the guitar around the house, and spent more time with the baby. In addition, he became "like a sex machine; morning and night, he was ever ready." Every time Sylvia walked into the room "there was a look in his eye." She had not seen anything like it in him since they were first married ten years before.

In fact, Sam was feeling so good that he told Sylvia that he no longer needed the new "vitamins." At that point, she felt constrained to explain to him why he was feeling so good and why he had better not stop the new pills. He took the news like a good sport, and acknowledged that he felt a release of positive energy. Now he says that he feels so good he will happily take St. John's wort for the rest of his life if that's what it takes to stay happy.

Matthew: Finding the Light at the End of the Tunnel

What would you do if you came home one day to find that your wife or husband had left you, had taken your two children away, and had cleared all the furniture out of the house? That's the situation that confronted Matthew one day when he returned home from his job as a security officer. Sometime later he completed one of my questionnaires about St. John's wort and allowed me to interview him in detail about his experiences. According to Matthew, there had been some difficulties in the marriage, but nothing that made him suspect that it was almost over. "She was so nice to me the night before she left," he mused wistfully, "it was as though she was giving me a going-away present." In fact, his wife had met another man and moved out of state to live with him, taking the two children with her.

For Matthew the loss was devastating. He had always been a sensitive person. Even as a young boy, he had always had "thin skin," feeling more stung than most by ordinary taunts from other boys in the school yard. Later, when it came time to date girls, he was always painfully aware when he did not have a girlfriend while others did. "I was always crushed by rejections," he recalls, "and would often be disinclined to try things because of fear of failure." He wondered whether his extreme sensitivity was somehow related to his pale, sun-sensitive skin, which went along with his red hair.

Being abandoned by his wife was one of the biggest blows of Matthew's life. He felt like a failure as a husband and a father and went into a profound depression that was to last for six years. During this time he felt like a bad person—if that were not the case, he reasoned, why would his wife have left him for another man? He couldn't sleep at night, as his mind "would race to places I wouldn't want it to go—back to the memories of being abandoned and betrayed by my wife." During the day, on the other hand, a cloud of exhaustion would overwhelm him when he was on his job and should have been attending to the security of the business for which he worked. He recalls how his eyelids "weighed a thousand pounds each" and he could barely stay awake. He craved junk foods—Big Macs, candy, doughnuts, chocolate ice cream, and cakes. His blood sugar became elevated and he needed medications to lower it.

Things became so bad that he felt as though he no longer

had any reason to live and he would ask himself, "What is this all for?" He went to the doctor for help, mindful that he had proved to be hypersensitive to almost all medications he had been given in the past. The doctor recommended Zoloft, but he suffered a serious allergic reaction after only a single dose. His eyes swelled shut, his heart "raced a hundred miles per hour," and he had nightmares and hallucinations.

Shortly after this experience, his mother saw a television program in which the benefits of St. John's wort were discussed and she suggested that he try it. Recognizing his sensitivity to medications, Matthew began by taking one 300-mg St. John's wort tablet per day. He felt some relief from the very first day and the improvement continued over the subsequent two months, by which time his depression had lifted completely. His sleep improved and even though the duration of sleep decreased, he "seemed to get more out of it," and felt more rested and alert during the day. His energy level "was boosted back to its normal level."

Matthew has returned to his old passion, music, and has begun to play his guitar again. For a long time, he'd forgotten that music even existed. He is overjoyed to have rediscovered it and sometimes catches himself singing. He has returned to church again, visiting different denominations to discuss religious ideas with different people. Along with his improved mental condition, Matthew's physical health is also better. Remarkably, given his sensitivity to medicines of all types, Matthew has experienced no side effects whatsoever on St. John's wort.

Even though his depression is over, Matthew recognizes that he is now faced with having to rebuild his life. "I am just beginning to see the light at the end of the tunnel," he observes, "but I'm not there yet." He plans to go to the gym and enroll in classes so that he can get a better job. He is even contemplating beginning to date again "without the old defeated attitude." He has begun to chat with an old high school sweetheart and is thinking of buying some new clothes and taking her out dancing.

He sums up his experiences with St. John's wort: "After six years of solid depression, of feeling crippled and at the edge of a cliff, ready to jump . . . all my ailments have subsided. I no longer feel any need for a medical professional. My faith has been restored. It's a miracle."

No doctors involved. No side effects. Complete remission of a chronic and disabling depression. Small wonder therefore that Matthew regards St. John's wort as a miracle herb that has given him back his life.

Mercedes: Lifting the Film of Dysthymia

Mercedes, another person who was good enough to complete one of my questionnaires, is a social worker in her early fifties. She makes a distinction between two different kinds of emotional suffering that she has experienced in the course of her life. The first type was "the remains of a difficult childhood," which it took her some time to sort out. But even after she was satisfied that she had taken care of the residue of her childhood, she was left with "a light film of dysthymia, which lasted for years and was probably inherited from my parents, both of whom suffered from depression." Dysthymia is a condition of chronic, persistent, low-grade depression.

As a result of her low mood, Mercedes would procrastinate, putting off unpleasant tasks such as housekeeping or paperwork in favor of activities she greatly preferred, such as knitting, crocheting, or playing with her birds and her dogs. Naturally introverted, she would withdraw in social situations, where she always felt as though she was holding back.

Mercedes decided to try St. John's wort, starting with 300 mg three times a day, because it was natural and she understood it to cause few side effects. It took at least five weeks to notice the herb's effect, and even then it was subtle, though palpable. She stopped procrastinating as much and was more outgoing in social situations. Her husband noted the change, remarking that her dark moodiness had lifted and that she now seemed lighter. She has experienced no side effects whatsoever, plans to continue to take the herbal antidepressant, and is interested in recommending it to several of her clients.

Although the condition of dysthymia is relatively mild, compared with some of the serious depressions one can find detailed in this book and elsewhere, it is by definition rather chronic. As such, it takes a serious toll on a person's capacity to enjoy life and be productive. Anything that can be done to relieve this chronic misery is greatly appreciated, and in this regard St. John's wort promises to be a blessing.

The stories of Matthew and Mercedes illustrate how versatile an antidepressant St. John's wort is, capable of bringing someone out of the dark depths of despair as in the case of Matthew, or of alleviating the milder and more subtle dysthymia that affected Mercedes. The dosages needed by these two individuals were quite different, with Matthew responding to one 300-mg tablet per day while Mercedes used the more conventional three-times-per-day dosing schedule. Optimal dosages of other types of antidepressant medications vary widely and there is no reason to suppose that this will prove to be different for St. John's wort. The size of the patient is not always a good guide to the best dosage, as these two cases illustrate, since Matthew, who is 6 feet tall and weighs 180 pounds, required only one third the dosage used by Mercedes, who is a small woman. Another difference between Matthew and Mercedes is the time course of action of the herbal antidepressant, from the almost immediate beneficial effects experienced by Matthew to the five-week lag before the treatment kicked in for Mercedes. Such observations indicate why it can be useful to experiment with different dosages for different people, and why it is important to persevere for several weeks before declaring a trial of St. John's wort to be a failure.

One exciting fact about antidepressants in general is that they are helpful in several conditions other than depression. People with disabling panic attacks, uncontrollable binge eating, and serious obsessions and compulsions have all benefited greatly from synthetic antidepressants. Early reports suggest that St. John's wort may have similar beneficial effects in some of these conditions and, once again, the absence of side effects makes the herbal remedy an alternative worth considering, as illustrated by the following stories.

Judy: I'm So Excited Because I Don't Want to Pull My Hair Out

Judy is a pretty woman of about thirty, whose regular features and cascade of straight auburn hair could easily be those of a model whose picture stares out at you from the window of a hair salon as a testament to the hairstylist's skills. What hardly anyone knows, though, is that for twenty-six years of her life, Judy would regularly pull out thousands of her hairs, leaving behind bald spots as wide as a golf ball. It was terribly embarrassing for her to look at these bald patches, and she would go to great lengths to conceal them with swatches of hair held down with barrettes or hairspray. In school she would stand at the back of the line so that no one would get close enough to her to see the bare patches. At the beach she would avoid putting her head under water for fear that the waves would sweep her hair to the side and expose the source of her embarrassment. Even when she met the man she was ultimately to marry, she resisted showering with him or letting him see the bald spots, and when it was finally impossible to conceal them from him anymore, she told him that they were the result of a bicycle accident.

Judy began to pull her hair out when she was thirteen years old, shortly after the death of her beloved grandmother, the person to whom she felt closer than anyone else in the world. She was sad and lonely and felt unable to talk about it to her family, who were all busy getting on with their own lives. One day in math class, she found herself pulling at her hair and felt comforted. That was the beginning of her secret addiction.

To add to her problem with hair pulling, Judy began to suffer from panic attacks when she was twenty-three. These occurred specifically when she went out to eat at restaurants. In the middle of a meal, her heart would start to pound, her hands would become sweaty, and she would be unable to swallow her food. Since eating out was one of her husband's favorite activities, this problem made her very unhappy. She took the anti-anxiety drug Xanax when she went out to dinner, which helped a little, but the panic persisted and she was still unable to enjoy the meal. After a while she began to anticipate with dread the prospect of dinner plans at a fancy restaurant and the persistent fear of having a panic attack felt worse than the panic itself.

In her thirties, Judy finally took her problem to a therapist and was given Prozac, a common type of treatment for panic attacks, but it made her feel unpleasantly jittery and she stopped taking it. Her husband's fortieth birthday was approaching and they had planned a trip to Bermuda to celebrate it. She knew that one of the highlights of the trip for him would be dining out at some of the fine restaurants on the island. She very much wanted to be able to enjoy that with him. At about that time she heard about St. John's wort and decided to give it a try.

Judy started on 300 mg per day of St. John's wort and felt a sense of calm within one day. Since she observed no side effects, she increased the dosage to 300 mg twice a day for the following five weeks. She and her husband went to Bermuda and, to her amazement, she was able to enjoy going to restaurants for the first time in many years. The panic attacks disappeared and she felt no need for Xanax any longer. Even more amazingly, she no longer had any desire to pull her hair out and she was even willing to show me the patches where fine hairs had begun to grow back. For the first time in twenty-six years, she no longer had bald patches that she had to cover or feel embarrassed about. She could barely contain her excitement at the fact that she no longer wanted to pull her hair out, and felt eager to share her story with fellow sufferers.

Trichotillomania

Judy's problem of compulsive hair pulling has a name—trichotillomania. It is surprisingly common among women who, like Judy, frequently conceal it from others by covering over the bald spots with hair. The condition is known to be very hard to treat, and antidepressants such as the selective serotonin reuptake inhibitors (SSRIs), which are so helpful in treating depression, panic disorder, bulimia, and obsessive-compulsive disorder, are much less successful in the treatment of trichotillomania. Behavioral strategies to reduce the ease of hair pulling, such as covering the head with a baseball cap or scarf, putting slippery styling mousse on it to make it harder to pull out the hairs, or wearing gloves may be of some help. But it is an uphill battle for those who are addicted to this activity. If St. John's wort proves to be helpful even in a small percentage of individuals affected by this painful and embarrassing condition, a great deal of suffering will be alleviated.

St. John's Wort and Panic Disorder

In addition to Judy, I have encountered another person whose panic-disorder symptoms appear to have been helped by St. John's wort. A twenty-five-year-old woman wrote to me from Germany that she had been plagued by episodes of anxiety, palpitations, vertigo, pressure in her chest, tension, and irritability—feelings she experienced especially intensely when in crowds and on car journeys. She treated these symptoms with St. John's wort with some success, finding that it helped her to deal better with stress in general as well as with the situations that triggered her anxiety.

Panic disorder is an extremely unpleasant condition characterized by brief but debilitating spells of anxiety that often come out of the blue and are accompanied by the very physical symptoms Judy reported. During panic attacks, the patient often feels trapped in the throes of a medical emergency and wracked by fears of impending death. Visits to the emergency room invariably yield negative results and a diagnosis of panic disorder is often made at that time. If the panic attacks continue unchecked, anxiety may become chronic as the person anticipates the next onslaught of the disorder. The final step in the progression of the disorder is a reluctance to leave home for fear that an attack will occur in an uncontrolled setting. This last symptom gives this disorder its alternate name—agorapho-bia, or fear of venturing into public places.

Since there appear to be certain pharmacological resem-blances between the mode of action of St. John's wort and that of other antidepressants, there is every reason to hope that the herbal antidepressant might also work for panic-disorder patients, just as it appears to have done for Judy and the other young woman described above. One cautionary note, however, if you are considering using the herb for this condition. Many people with panic disorder are extremely sensitive to all antide-pressants, becoming more anxious and jittery after receiving their first antidepressant tablets. It is therefore commonplace in using conventional antidepressants in the treatment of panic disorder to start with very low dosages and move the dosage up gradually as the patient becomes more able to tolerate the med-ication. After a while, it may be possible to raise the antidepres-sant dosage to conventional levels without undue discomfort to the patient. Following these general principles, I would suggest that anyone attempting to treat panic disorder with St. John's wort obtain it in the form of a liquid preparation known as a tincture, start treatment with no more than one tenth of the recommended number of drops per day, and move up from there (or down if even this low dose feels too much), being guided by levels of side effects in determining the dosing pro-gression. Once a comfortable therapeutic dosage has been reached, I recommend switching to the Kira brand of St. John's wort, the brand that has been shown to be effective in the largest number of research studies on depressed patients.

As these stories indicate, we are just beginning to recognize the full scope of St. John's wort's therapeutic potential. As more research accumulates, we will be able to answer with a greater degree of precision questions about when to try the herb and how to prioritize it in choosing the best treatment for a given patient or condition. Until that happens, though, it is important to recognize that the herb is a real option, to be considered alongside other therapeutic options, in the treatment of a wide variety of emotional disturbances.

4

SCIENCE AND ST. JOHN'S WORT

What the Research Shows

Even though research is still going on, the available data show that hypericum extract is clinically effective as an antidepressant drug and that it probably works by biochemical mechanisms not so very different from the mechanisms of action of the tricyclics or the SSRIs. We feel that these findings are important enough to be communicated and interesting enough to stimulate further research.

—Dr. WALTER E. MÜLLER, UNIVERSITY OF
FRANKFURT, AND Dr. SIEGFRIED KASPER,
UNIVERSITY OF VIENNA, *PHARMACOPSYCHIATRY*,
1997

The modern era of research into St. John's wort was ushered in by the former German Federal Health Agency, which set up Commission E to investigate the evidence for the beneficial effects of the many herbal remedies in general use in Germany and to find out which of these herbs appeared to be safe and effective for one condition or another. Commission E came out with its report in 1984 and identified approximately three hundred herbs for which such evidence existed. Shortly after that, certain German pharmaceutical companies targeted some of these herbs as worthy of particular research attention, and St. John's wort was one of these targeted herbs.

Research into a new treatment, such as St. John's wort for depression, usually develops in predictable ways. One needs to establish whether the treatment actually works, who benefits most from it, what dosages are appropriate, and for how long treatment should be continued. Its safety needs to be assured and side effects need to be documented. And only once the treatment is regarded as safe and effective does attention usually turn to how the treatment actually works. Research on St. John's wort is ongoing, but so far it has taken these expected directions. In this chapter I summarize the state of the art of research on this herbal antidepressant.

Is St. John's Wort an Effective Antidepressant?

The only studies of the efficacy of St. John's wort conducted to date were done in Europe. These studies initially came to the attention of the U.S. medical community when an issue of the *Journal of Geriatric Psychiatry and Neurology* was devoted to hypericum in 1994, and later when the highly regarded *British Medical Journal* published an article reviewing the data on all well-conducted clinical studies of St. John's wort for depression that had been published at the time of the review. This review, known technically as a meta-analysis, combined several small studies in order to determine whether certain general conclusions could be drawn from the available data.

In their meta-analysis, K. Linde and colleagues addressed three simple questions:

- Is hypericum more effective than a placebo?

- Is it as effective as standard antidepressant treatments?

- Does it have fewer side effects than standard antidepressant treatments?

In order to increase their chances of reaching valid conclusions, these researchers included in their meta-analysis only those studies that used state-of-the-art methods in their design and in the analysis of their data.

Interestingly, when Linde and colleagues used only conventional computerized searches of the medical literature, they located fewer than a third of those clinical trials that they ultimately chose to include. The other two thirds of the studies had been published in alternative medicine journals that were not readily available to mainstream medical practitioners. The experience of these researchers reflects the division separating herbal and conventional medicine that has been so prominent until recently and that persists to a considerable extent even at the present time. Almost all studies were published in German, an indication of how the recent developments in herbal medicine have come predominantly from the German-speaking world. Finally, the authors had to go through many revisions before the prestigious mainstream *British Medical Journal* was willing to publish the review.

Altogether, the authors analyzed 23 randomized trials involving 1,757 patients suffering from mild to moderate depression.

- In thirteen trials of hypericum versus a placebo, Linde and colleagues found hypericum to be clearly superior to the placebo, yielding a response rate of 55 percent as compared with 22 percent for the placebo treatment.

- In three trials of hypericum versus standard antidepressants, the two treatments were very similar. But when side effects were compared, hypericum emerged as the clear winner, with approximately 20 percent of the hypericum group reporting side effects as compared with about 53 percent of those taking standard antidepressants.

  Several studies reviewed by the researchers used combinations of St. John's wort and valerian, an herbal sedative. I have excluded these studies from the present discussion, though their results were consistent with those that used St. John's wort alone.

- Linde and colleagues concluded rather persuasively that hypericum is superior to a placebo in the treatment of mild to moderate depression and that it has a very benign side-effect profile.

The evidence was less clear-cut when it came to comparing the relative benefits of St. John's wort with other antidepressants because adequate comparative studies between herbal and synthetic antidepressants have not been performed. Those studies of this type that have been performed to date have been faulted because the dosages of synthetic antidepressants that were used were lower than those often used in clinical practice.

The conclusions of the meta-analysis of studies on St. John's wort can be called into question for a few reasons. First, it is possible that negative studies, namely those that failed to show any advantage of hypericum over a placebo, might never have been published, thereby exaggerating the beneficial effects of the herb. Second, since most of the studies used a narrow dosage range of hypericum (between 600 and 900 mg per day), we do not have a good understanding of the full range of dosages that might prove beneficial. Observing a relationship between dosage and effect is one way in which researchers become persuaded that an antidepressant really works and learn how best to administer it. Third, since most of the published studies are in German, English-speaking experts have not yet had a chance to evaluate them fully. Finally, the different studies used different herbal preparations and methods as well as different types of patients. These differences limit the validity of pooling together the results.

Clearly, there is room for more research on the efficacy of St. John's wort, especially into questions of who would best benefit from hypericum versus conventional antidepressants, how best to regulate dosage, and how to combine hypericum with conventional antidepressants. To date, there have been no head-to-head comparisons between St. John's wort and the SSRIs. Such a comparison is part of the design of the multicenter U.S. study currently being planned under the aegis of the National Institute of Mental Health. It is important to compare these two types of antidepressants, since at present the SSRIs are more commonly used. In practice, both doctor and patient may often wish to choose between them in deciding how to initiate the treatment of depression.

There have been no long-term studies of the antidepressant effects of St. John's wort but, in this regard, the herbal antidepressant is no different from many of the conventional antidepressants for which long-term studies are lacking.

While many questions about the advantages of St. John's wort have yet to be resolved to the satisfaction of scientists, for the person seeking relief from the painful symptoms of depression, they are of much less importance than the fundamental question, "Does the herbal antidepressant work?" In my view this question has already been answered with a resounding yes.

Is St. John's Wort Helpful in Severe Depression?

Most research into St. John's wort has involved patients with mild to moderate depression. To date there has been only one study that has addressed the question of whether St. John's wort works for more serious depression. Clinical reports from Germany in the early part of the century, which I detail more fully later in this book, suggest that the herbal remedy might be helpful in severe as well as in milder cases. In recent times, Dr. Ernst-Ulrich Vorbach and colleagues in Germany conducted a multicenter study of 209 severely depressed patients, of whom 38 were hospitalized at the time of the study. They used a higher dosage of hypericum than had been used in the studies of mild to moderate depressions (1,800 mg, or six pills per day, as opposed to 900 mg, or three pills) and compared this with imipramine, an old, standard tricyclic antidepressant. While the antidepressant effects of these two treatments were very similar, far fewer side effects were reported by those receiving hypericum than by those receiving imipramine (23 versus 41 percent). This study suggests that there may indeed be a role for hypericum in the treatment of severe depression, though more studies on such patients are clearly needed before St. John's wort can be used with any confidence as a first-line treatment in profoundly depressed individuals.

As I note later, there is one study that suggests hypericum to be of value in seasonal affective disorder (SAD), though no one has properly researched how best to combine the herbal remedy with light therapy.

Is Hypericum Safe? What Are Its Side Effects?

Extensive usage of St. John's wort in Europe over the past decade strongly suggests that the herb is both safe and well tolerated when high-quality brands are used in the dosages commonly prescribed.

One of the most comprehensive surveys of the side effects of hypericum was performed by Dr. Helmut Woelk and colleagues in Germany, who monitored 3,250 patients being treated with hypericum by 663 private practitioners. The vast majority of these patients were considered to be mildly or moderately depressed. Interestingly, in this survey, only 30 percent of patients were considered to have improved as a result of their treatment, approximately half the percentage of responders reported in the far more reliable data base of the meta-analysis mentioned above. This might have been due to the lower dosages of hypericum used in general clinical practice as opposed to the 900 mg per day used in most of the controlled studies.

Of all the patients monitored, only 2.4 percent reported side effects and only 1.5 percent stopped their treatment because of side effects.

The most common side effects reported were:

- gastrointestinal irritations
- allergic reactions
- restlessness

Each of these side effects occurred with a frequency of less than 1 percent. These figures were again far lower than those in the *British Medical Journal* report where 20 percent of patients on hypericum in one set of studies and 4 percent of patients in another set complained of side effects while being treated with hypericum.

Skin Sensitivity

One special side-effect concern that has been raised in regard to St. John's wort is whether it increases the sensitivity of the skin to sunlight in a potentially harmful way. Toxic sun-sensitive skin reactions in cattle have drawn attention to the plant for decades, raising questions as to whether such reactions could occur in humans as well. Apparently, not to a troublesome degree in dosages that are ordinarily used, according to Dr. Jürgen Brockmöller and colleagues in Germany, who have used volunteers to test the effects of simulated sunlight. They gave one set of study subjects four times the ordinary dosage of hypericum in a single dose and another set of subjects 600 mg (two pills) per day for two weeks. They found only very slight increases in the tendency of the skin to redden or tan under both conditions and no evidence of any toxic reactions. What this means is that if you are on St. John's wort, you need to be a bit more careful about exposure to sunlight, as you are likely to redden or tan a bit more than usual. Incidentally, such side effects are common with many other antidepressants and nonpsychiatric medications such as certain antibiotics and Retin-A as well.

How Does St. John's Wort Work?

Before we try to answer this question, it is important to concede up front that researchers do not know for sure how any antidepressant works. But we have a strong suspicion that the first step in the action of most commonly used antidepressants is to influence the way in which nerve signals are transmitted from one nerve cell, or neuron, to another. The brain consists of millions of neurons, which communicate with one another at synapses, points at which they are in close proximity but do not actually touch. Neural signals pass along the transmitting neuron in the form of electrical impulses until they reach the synapse, where they are converted to chemical signals that stimulate the receiving neuron, where they are once again converted into electrical signals. Normal transmission of electrical signals along neuronal pathways is necessary for the proper maintenance of all brain-regulated functions, including the control of mood, sleep, eating, thinking, and the other basic processes that are disrupted in depression.

The chemical transmission of the signal at the synapse involves the release of specific nerve chemical messengers, or neurotransmitters, that are housed in little pockets or vesicles in the transmitting neuron at the synapse, where they act on specific receptors on the surface of the receiving neuron. After they have communicated their chemical messages, the neurotransmitters are taken back up into the transmitting neuron again, which terminates the nerve signal. After being taken back up into the transmitting neuron, the neurotransmitters are broken down by an enzyme called monoamine oxidase, or MAO.

The reuptake of released neurotransmitters that follows a nerve signal is handled by special transporter proteins attached to the surface of the transmitting neuron. The transporter proteins for the neurotransmitters involved in synaptic transmission have been the focus of considerable attention because most commonly used antidepressants inhibit the reuptake of neurotransmitters by these proteins, a step that is thought to be the initial action that sets in motion a cascade of effects ultimately responsible for reversing the symptoms of depression. Inhibiting the reuptake of a neurotransmitter causes it to remain in the synaptic cleft where it can exert its effect for longer than would be the case in the absence of an antidepressant. This is thought to initiate the salutary effects of antidepressants on mood.

Different neurons use different types of neurotransmitters to conduct their messages. Those neurotransmitters that have been most intensively studied are serotonin, norepinephrine, and dopamine. These neurotransmitters are thought to be important in regulating different aspects of mood. Serotonin, for example, is thought to be involved in feelings of satisfaction and contentment and norepinephrine with feelings of alertness and activation, while dopamine is thought to mediate social interactions. All of these functions can be disturbed in depressed people. One of the major ways in which antidepressants differ from one another stems from the relative potency with which they inhibit the reuptake of these different neurotransmitters. These differences affect their side-effect profiles and probably their therapeutic effects as well.

Older tricyclic antidepressants were rather unselective in their effects, affecting many different types of receptors, including those that are not thought to have anything to do with depression. For this reason, they caused several undesirable side effects. When the newer family of antidepressants, including the enormously popular Prozac and Zoloft, were introduced, their major attraction was that they selectively affected serotonin reuptake without affecting other neurotransmitters to anywhere near the same degree: hence their generic name, selective serotonin reuptake inhibitors (SSRIs). Another antidepressant commonly used in the United States, bupropion, or Wellbutrin, is thought to act more selectively on dopamine and norepinephrine. Our understanding of the effects of antidepressants on neuronal function comes largely from experiments performed on animal brains, though the results are believed to be applicable to the intact human brain as well.

Given the central role that the inhibition of reuptake of neurotransmitters appears to play in the action of other antidepressants, it was logical to ask whether St. John's wort might have such effects as well, and that is precisely what Dr. Walter E. Müller and colleagues in Germany set out to study. They found that an extract of St. John's wort is capable of inhibiting the reuptake of all three neurotransmitters mentioned above—serotonin, norepinephrine, and dopamine.

If these findings turn out to be correct, it may mean that St. John's wort has a unique pharmacological profile, affecting serotonin like the SSRIs, and dopamine and norepinephrine like Wellbutrin, but not the receptors responsible for the unpleasant side effects associated with the older antidepressants. Patients with depression or other conditions might feel more cheerful and calmer as a result of the effects on serotonin, more alert and energetic as a result of the effects on nor-epinephrine, and more inclined to reach out to others as a result of the effects on dopamine. My own clinical impressions are in keeping with these research findings, as St. John's wort appears to be uniquely beneficial and well tolerated in certain individuals, some of whom I describe elsewhere in this book.

As far as side effects are concerned, clinical experience suggests that for some people the newer SSRIs appear to cause more bothersome sexual side effects than do the older antidepressants, which affected both serotonin and norepinephrine transmission. The balanced profile of neurotransmitter reuptake inhibition found with St. John's wort may explain why many people appear to experience fewer sexual side effects on the herbal antidepressant than they do on the SSRIs.

Is St. John's Wort a Monoamine Oxidase Inhibitor (MAOI)?

Early reports suggested that St. John's wort might act as a monoamine oxidase inhibitor (MAOI). As I mentioned above, MAO is the enzyme responsible for breaking down neurotransmitters after they have been taken back up into the transmitting neuron at the synapse. If this enzyme is inhibited, the concentrations of these neurotransmitters increase in the synapse, which is believed to be the way in which a group of antidepressants, the MAO inhibitors (or MAOIs), such as Nardil or Parnate, exert their beneficial effects. A major problem with these drugs, however, is that they inhibit MAO in parts of the body other than the brain, most important, in the bowel, where the enzyme is normally responsible for detoxifying chemicals contained in ordinary foods such as yellow cheese and red wine. As a consequence, if someone on an MAO inhibitor should eat one of these prohibited foods, a serious toxic reaction can result, with a marked and sometimes dangerous elevation of blood pressure. In addition, there is a potential for dangerous interactions between MAO inhibitors and other drugs such as the SSRIs.

If St. John's wort were indeed an MAO inhibitor of any

potency, this would seriously limit its usefulness. The good news is that the researchers in Frankfurt, Germany, found that St. John's wort is *not* an MAO inhibitor to any significant degree. These findings suggest that there is no reason for those taking the herbal antidepressant to avoid any particular foods, such as cheese, which can be harmful to those taking MAOIs. In addition, there is no good evidence that it is any more harmful to combine St. John's wort with other antidepressants than it would be to combine synthetic antidepressants with one another, which is standard practice in the medical treatment of depression. Of course, if antidepressants are to be combined, it is always important that this be done carefully and under the supervision of a physician; this applies equally well to St. John's wort as to synthetic antidepressants. In addition, you should not combine an MAOI, such as Nardil or Parnate, with St. John's wort, just as you would avoid combining an MAOI with most other antidepressants.

Delayed Brain Effects of St. John's Wort Resemble Those Seen with Conventional Antidepressants

No one knows for sure why it generally takes antidepressants, including St. John's wort, several weeks to produce their effects. The effects on reuptake of neurotransmitters seen following administration of most antidepressants are immediate and are therefore unlikely to be a complete explanation of clinical effects that take weeks to unfold. Current thinking holds that effects of antidepressants on reuptake of neurotransmitters may be just the first in a cascade of biochemical steps necessary for reversing the symptoms of depression. Certain brain changes in receptors thought to be relevant to depression have been observed to occur a few weeks after antidepressant treatment is started. Because the timing of these changes corresponds to the time lag required for the antidepressant's clinical effects to kick in, they may provide an explanation as to how the antidepressants are working. Interestingly, delayed brain changes in rats similar to those seen following administration of conventional antidepressant treatments have also been found to occur a few weeks after administration of St. John's wort. This is another piece of biochemical evidence linking the beneficial effects of the herbal antidepressant to those of conventional synthetic ones.

Research Still to Be Done

In addition to continuing the lines of research already started, and summarized above, other important research directions should be explored. I will mention a few of these.

1. Effects in Other Psychiatric Conditions

Antidepressants, such as the earlier tricyclics and the selective serotonin reuptake inhibitors, have been found to help individuals with psychiatric conditions other than depression. These include panic disorder, bulimia, anorexia, obsessive-compulsive disorder, and social phobia. Future research should be geared toward exploring the potential benefits of the herbal remedy on these conditions.

People with panic disorder are overwhelmed by attacks of anxiety, associated with pounding of the heart, shortness of breath, and sweating, often accompanied by a sense of impending doom. Antidepressants, if used on a regular basis, have been found to forestall these attacks. I have observed a few people whose panic attacks have responded very well to St. John's wort and it seems likely that the herb will prove to be a valuable alternative to conventional antidepressants for the treatment of this condition.

Those with social phobia, that painful dread of public humiliation that paralyzes people in a variety of social situations, can respond well to antidepressants, particularly those that affect the neurotransmitter dopamine. Dopamine systems in the brain mediate many functions, which include the inclination to interact with others. As St. John's wort appears to affect dopamine, along with other neurotransmitters, it is logical to consider the potential value of the herb for social phobia.

As I have described, some shy and reticent people have clearly become more outgoing and assertive after starting St. John's wort. A more systematic trial of the use of the herb for this condition would be well worthwhile.

According to American Indian folk healers, St. John's wort can be useful for treating bed-wetting, a problem that is distressing both to the children who experience it and their parents. This condition, also known as enuresis, has been reported to respond to one of the older antidepressants, imipramine. Just as St. John's wort exhibits some of the other beneficial effects of imipramine, so it might also prove useful in the treatment of enuresis.

The neurotransmitter serotonin seems to be disturbed in people with bulimia and obsessive-compulsive disorder. As St. John's wort appears to affect the transmission of nerve signals involving serotonin, it is possible that it might also help people with these conditions. People with bulimia tend to binge voraciously and frequently induce vomiting afterward, while those with obsessive-compulsive disorder suffer from a variety of disturbing thoughts that preoccupy them, along with compulsive behaviors such as checking on things, washing their hands, or pulling out their hair. I have described one young woman whose distressing hair pulling has been alleviated by St. John's wort. I believe that we have only just begun to recognize the scope of this herb in treating this and other conditions. These are areas ripe for future research. Until that research is conducted, however, St. John's wort may be considered as a real treatment option for these conditions if, for any reason, standard treatments appear undesirable or problematic.

2. Effects on Wound Healing and As an Antiviral Agent

Reports on the beneficial effects of St. John's wort for the healing of wounds go back almost two thousand years and predate its use as an antidepressant. Nevertheless, in modern times, research into this particular application of the herb has lagged behind its psychiatric uses and awaits proper study. There are suggestions that extracts of St. John's wort may have beneficial effects for those infected with viruses such as HIV and herpes. Clinical trials are needed to determine the efficacy of this herb for these conditions. There are other treatments, however, with proven efficacy against such viral infections and they should certainly be used before using an experimental treatment. Given the tendency for viruses to develop resistances to a variety of medications, however, the possibility of a new weapon, derived from nature's arsenal, to fight these deadly killers is an exciting prospect that awaits further exploration.

3. Further Understanding of the Pharmacological Effects of St. John's Wort

Our understanding of how St. John's wort exerts its beneficial effects and how it influences relevant biological systems is in its early phases. We do not even know for sure which of the many biologically active compounds in St. John's wort extracts are responsible for its antidepressant actions. Researchers suspect that the substances hypericin and pseudohypericin, formerly supposed to be the most active ingredients in this regard, may not be responsible at all. Instead attention has turned to another substance, hyperforin, as the one most likely to be the active antidepressant ingredient. Müller and colleagues have shown that the effects of hypericum extracts on the reuptake of neurotransmitters are similar to those of this ingredient, hyperforin, used in its pure form. Clearly, the last word is not in on this subject, but it would be very useful to know what the active ingredients are so that they can be distilled into a more potent or specific essence. It would also be very advantageous to know how St. John's wort is metabolized and how it may influence the metabolism of other medications that a patient may require along with the herbal remedy. Such information is lacking at this time, and although no conspicuous interactions with other drugs are uncommon, more specific data in this area would be very welcome.

In summary, we have strong evidence that St. John's wort works well for a wide variety of depressed patients and that it is very well tolerated. As is the nature of science, each new piece of information raises new questions. For the researcher, these are important questions to ask and to answer, but for the person suffering from depression, who stands to benefit right now from the herbal antidepressant, many of these questions are of secondary importance to the observation that the herb works for a diversity of problems in many, many people.

5

SWITCHING FROM CONVENTIONAL ANTIDEPRESSANTS TO ST. JOHN'S WORT AND USING MEDICATION COMBINATIONS

Although no scientific studies comparing St. John's wort to the most commonly used antidepressants, the SSRIs, have been conducted to date, many people who have switched to St. John's wort clearly prefer the herbal antidepressant. Some who have made the switch point out the following advantages of St. John's wort:

- fewer sexual side effects

- less weight gain

- less difficulty thinking and remembering

- no feelings of being dull and lifeless

- fewer gastrointestinal upsets

These advantages are illustrated in some of the case studies described below. It will be interesting to see whether formal studies corroborate the observations of these people. In the meantime, however, those who are experiencing side effects on their current antidepressants may wish to discuss with their physician whether it makes sense to consider switching to St. John's wort.

One young woman wrote to me with the following comments, which were typical of many responses I received to my questionnaire. She had used St. John's wort for the previous nine months to treat her symptoms of depression and anxiety and reported: "St. John's wort has helped me an incredible amount without producing the side effects I experienced with Prozac, such as decreased interest in sex and weight gain. It's been a miracle." The story that follows illustrates another potential advantage of the herbal remedy.

Fiona: Thinking More Clearly on St. John's Wort

Fiona is a sixty-year-old social worker and mother of three grown children who has been troubled by depression and mood fluctuations for years. Her depressive symptoms have often seemed more physical than emotional. During her depressions, she would become fatigued, her arms and legs would feel heavy, her eyelids would begin to droop, preventing her from being able to read, and she would feel "kind of sad and tired," wanting to sleep much of the time. To some extent these problems may have been related to a condition of adrenal failure, known as Addison's disease, from which Fiona suffers. The steroid replacement that is necessary to control her medical condition has been partly responsible for causing Fiona's moods to fluctuate. Because of these mood variations she has never been able to rely on her ability to cope and has chosen not to work at her profession.

Fiona had been on 20 mg a day of Prozac for six or seven years. Although she credits Prozac with lifting her out of her depression, it left her with a "dazed view of the world." Things did not feel "quite real." Her mind was not clear and she would forget things. Her reactions were delayed and it was hard to keep up with a conversation even though she had previously been very sociable and outgoing.

Fiona's doctor wondered to what degree her problems with thinking were due to the Prozac and stopped the medication in order to find out. She soon became depressed again, at which time he started her on St. John's wort (500 to 750 mg per day).

Within two weeks her mood picked up. Her thinking was clearer and she was able to read again. She rates the antidepressant effect of the St. John's wort on a par with that of Prozac, but she feels that she is now "part of the world again." With her newfound clarity, she has restarted therapy, and is contacting friends and having lunch with them. She has even initiated "play groups for adults," where friends come over simply to do fun things like painting or throwing medicine balls around. These get-togethers remind her of the "co-operative games of the sixties." "I never got to play them then," she observes, "and I want to play them now."

Less Abdominal Discomfort on St. John's Wort

James, a fifty-year-old professional, wrote to me as follows:

> I have had one form or another of depression for over ten years. My depression has greatly affected my life in many ways. Most notably, my relationship with my wife suffered and my relationship and reactions to daily work circumstances have been greatly and negatively affected. Many of my attempts to deal with my depression failed.

James described how he first underwent six months of psychotherapy, which was of no help, followed by a course of Paxil, which helped his depression slightly but caused him chronic diarrhea, a liability far greater than its minimal benefit in relieving his depression. At one point, when he broke his foot, this side effect became even more inconvenient as he had difficulty getting to the bathroom on time. He decided to discontinue the medication and his depression returned in full force.

After doing some research on St. John's wort, James decided to take the herb on his own and within six weeks of starting to take 300 mg three times a day, his feelings of depression began to subside. "My depression is now manageable, and

I would have to say almost nonexistent," he concludes. "I hope St. John's wort remains available without a prescription and that the . . . medical professionals do not attempt to 'prescriptionize' it. . . . I hope my short personal history regarding my depression and travels toward St. John's wort will help keep it available to the general public."

Better Sex on St. John's Wort

Greater enjoyment of sex and improved sexual functioning are among the most commonly reported contrasts between the effects of St. John's wort and those of the selective serotonin reuptake inhibitors (SSRIs) such as Prozac, Zoloft, and Paxil. Although some of the literature on the SSRIs reports very low levels of sexual side effects (for example, less than 1 percent for Prozac and 2.5 percent for Zoloft), any clinician who prescribes these medications will tell you that these figures are gross underestimates. One survey of patients on Prozac reported that about one third of all successfully treated patients reported some form of sexual problem. There is no evidence that other SSRIs are any better in this regard. Considering the importance of sex in the lives of many (if not most) people, it is worth paying attention to the improvement in the sex lives of people who have switched from an SSRI to the herbal antidepressant.

The degree of sexual problems experienced with the SSRIs is quite variable. In some people the sexual side effects of the SSRIs can be extremely marked. For example, they may cause impotence in men or complete inability to have an orgasm in women. In my experience, Paxil is one of the worst culprits. I recall once striking up a conversation with a fellow passenger on an airplane who, as soon as he heard I was a psychiatrist, asked me what I thought of Paxil, the antidepressant that had been prescribed for him. I told him that I had had little luck with the drug, especially with men because of their frequent complaints about sexual side effects. "Ah," he exclaimed with delight, "so that's what's doing it to me! I'm going to stop it at once." I suggested that he consult his doctor first.

Depressed people generally have a diminished interest in sex to start with, and any antidepressant, by reversing the symptoms of depression, may improve the level of interest and overall drive to connect with others sexually as well as socially. Initially, people are so grateful to be free of their depression that any sexual side effects they might experience may seem like a small price to pay for feeling better. After a while, though, the side effects become less and less acceptable as they begin to take a toll on the person's relationships and impair his or her quality of life.

Sexual side effects of the SSRIs can involve decreases in sexual interest, arousal, or subtle changes in the experience of sex. A colleague of mine, for example, who was previously on Zoloft and is now taking St. John's wort, described how on Zoloft he had been able to function sexually but the orgasms just did not feel as good. "On Zoloft," he recalls, "I was still interested in sex and my erections were fine, but it took me longer to reach orgasm, and when I did, the arc of the orgasm was slower and more protracted and did not reach its previously satisfying level of intensity. I am glad to say that on St. John's wort my orgasms are back to normal again."

Given our best understanding that St. John's wort probably works at least in part by inhibiting the reuptake of serotonin, the biological mechanism believed to be responsible for the sexual side effects of the SSRIs, some sexual side effects might be expected to be reported as the herbal antidepressant is more widely used. I have already encountered two people who claim some alteration in libido and sexual pleasure on St. John's wort, albeit to a lesser degree than on the SSRIs. Such problems may occur with more frequency if people push the dosage of the herb above 900 mg per day as I predict many will in their attempts to explore the full range of the herb's efficacy. Nevertheless, St. John's wort appears to be far less disruptive of sexual enjoyment and functioning than the SSRIs. This may be due to the influence of St. John's wort on neurotransmitters other than serotonin, as opposed to the SSRIs, which act almost exclusively on serotonin transmission.

It is important to remember that a slight decrease in sexual enjoyment may be an acceptable trade-off in exchange for being free of the painful symptoms of depression. One man whose depressions had been successfully treated with Prozac for the previous two years switched to St. John's wort after seeing a television program about it. Two weeks after the switch he wrote to me that "the ol' sex drive has come back with a vengeance . . . my wife is thrilled." Several months later, however, I checked on how he was doing and learned that his depression had recurred and that he had developed panic attacks, which resulted in his returning to conventional antidepressants.

It must be acknowledged that no medication, herbal or otherwise, is right for everyone. Some people will no doubt end up doing better on synthetic antidepressants than on St. John's wort, whereas others, such as the people described in this chapter, did better with the herbal remedy. It is a great comfort, however, for those suffering from unpleasant or even disabling emotional conditions to be aware that another treatment option is now available to them.

Switching from a Conventional Antidepressant to St. John's Wort

Considering the buzz surrounding the new herbal antidepressant, it is likely that many people will choose to switch from the conventional antidepressant they are already taking and try the herbal remedy instead. Let me repeat a few suggested guidelines if you should decide to do so.

- Do not switch just for the sake of switching. If you are doing well on a particular antidepressant, with minimal side effects, it makes good sense to leave well enough alone. If this is not the case, a switch is worth considering.
- Involve your doctor in the process (after all, someone must be prescribing the antidepressant).
- Switch gradually, overlapping the two medications in the transition phase.

- Monitor your progress carefully to ensure that you do not suffer a relapse.
- Be sure to report promptly to you doctor any side effects that may occur during this transition. In rare instances, people have experienced confusion, overexcitement, or restlessness when on combinations of St. John's wort and other antidepressants.
- Be open-minded about returning to your previous treatment sooner rather than later if the switch does not appear to be working.

The following four stories describe successful transitions from a conventional to an herbal antidepressant. The first person was referred to me for consultation; the second is someone whom I treated years ago; the other two are currently under my care.

Henry: The Doctor Who Thought He Was a Fraud

Henry is a research physician in his late forties who was referred to me for consultation about the possibility of including St. John's wort in his treatment regimen. He has a very long history of suffering, going all the way to his childhood, and has struggled with severe depression for the past eighteen years.

As a child, Henry was excessively timid, a trait that was reinforced by his parents, who were rigid disciplinarians. He was expected to be "a good boy," to toe the line at all times, and to recognize that his parents were always right. Any suggestion that this might not be so would elicit stony, quiet anger from his mother and attacks of terrifying rage from his father.

Henry drew some solace from his academic studies, in which he always excelled, and easily whizzed through medical school, taking all the prizes at graduation day. Shortly after graduating, he fell in love and got married. So far, so good.

When he started his residency, Henry began to be plagued by waves of self-doubt regarding his clinical skills and believed himself to be a fraud, an inadequate physician posing as a competent one. These nagging concerns, which had no basis in reality, turned each workday into a nightmare of fear and anxiety that "the truth" would be exposed, that he would be publicly humiliated, and that his career would end in catastrophic ruin.

After his residency, Henry embarked on his lifelong dream of becoming a researcher. That is when his depressions began in earnest. He regarded his supervisor as a father figure and, like his father, the man was stern, exacting, and "always right." Henry's research went badly, and because the supervisor was a famous researcher, the failure to make progress was blamed entirely on Henry, who became increasingly depressed. He suffered from severe early morning waking and feelings of terror, and began to have panic attacks at work.

Henry recognized that this research environment was toxic, wanted to relocate, and succeeded in finding another position, but, at the last minute, his supervisor asked him to stay and once again, out of fear of taking the chance of being exposed as a fraud in his new position, he agreed to stay. The research remained unproductive, his relationship with his supervisor deteriorated, and his feelings of depression, failure, and worthlessness increased over the days, weeks, and months.

His wife, who remained supportive at all times, was unsuccessful in persuading him to seek psychiatric help. Finally, out of frustration, she sought it out herself. At that point, Henry agreed to seek out a therapist, who helped him start to understand the impact his upbringing had had on his ability to function as an adult. As a result of the therapy, Henry became enraged and his depression deepened. The therapist, a member of the "old school" of psychiatry, refused to medicate the depression, claiming that it would interfere with the therapeutic process. When Henry insisted on medication, the therapist placed him on an inadequately low dosage of one of the older antidepressants.

Shortly afterward the therapist went on a sabbatical and Henry was referred to another psychiatrist whose major expertise was in the use of antidepressant medications. For the next thirteen years, this man treated Henry with a succession of antidepressants, together with supportive therapy. In those days, before the arrival of the SSRIs, all available antidepressants were used, including the older tricyclic antidepressants, lithium carbonate, trazodone, Wellbutrin, and the MAOIs, which are often regarded as the big guns, to be brought out when nothing else works. During this period, in response to Henry's unremitting symptoms, the psychiatrist sent him to a number of different prestigious psychopharmacologists for consultation, but to no avail. On the contrary, he continued to be plagued by frequent attacks of suicidal feelings and had actually developed a plan for how he would kill himself in such a way as to make it appear as though it was not a suicide. Had it not been for his wife and children, Henry believes he might have followed through on this plan.

Finally, Henry found a psychopharmacologist who emphasized the importance of his anxiety to his problem and persuaded Henry to take the anti-anxiety medication Klonopin for his panic attacks. At the same time Henry was put on Zoloft. He noticed a dramatic improvement over a two-week period, and over the course of the next few years he became less depressed and anxious. His panic attacks disappeared and he became increasingly productive at work. At the same time, this treatment unleashed another wave of rage directed against his supervisor and a number of people he believed had not treated him properly during his years of depression.

He stayed on this treatment for five years and was relatively satisfied with the results until he began to believe that he was still chronically, though subclinically, depressed. He was continually tired, slept ten to twelve hours a day, and had little energy for anything other than his work. His wife, who had continued to tolerate his depressed state, now began to complain that he was totally immersed in his work, unavailable to her, and insufficiently helpful around the house. He entered therapy again and brought his wife along with him so that she could relay her concerns to the therapist. Now he was able to benefit from the therapy, which focused on neurotic issues that continued to arise. He still became excessively angry at old friends and coworkers and obsessed continually about one or another of his personal interactions, to the detriment of his work and personal life. In addition, he recognized that his sexual functioning had become abnormal in that he had difficulty reaching orgasm and derived little sensual pleasure from doing so. Henry had been willing to tolerate this side effect, which started within weeks of beginning Zoloft, accepting it as a reasonable trade-off for his improved mood. After all this time, however, it was becoming increasingly bothersome to him.

After reading about my interest in St. John's wort, Henry was referred to me for consultation and I suggested that he add St. John's wort to his current mix of medications, which consisted of very high dosages of Zoloft, Wellbutrin, and the anti-anxiety medication Klonopin. As always, I suggested that he add the St. John's wort gradually, and he began with one tablet (300 mg) a day for about three weeks. He noticed an effect within a week, which he could only describe as a newfound "joie de vivre." Over the next few weeks, under my direction, he continued to increase the dosage of St. John's wort and decrease the dosage of Wellbutrin and Zoloft. During this period he noticed a progressive increase in energy and well-being, a dissipation of his obsessive thoughts, and improved sexual functioning. As a scientist, he began to become more of a risk-taker, more imaginative, and his work benefited enormously from these new developments. His wife noticed the differences in him within a few weeks of his starting the herbal antidepressant.

Currently Henry is on a total dosage of 1,200 mg of St. John's wort per day (two tablets twice a day). He is off all other antidepressants and has held on to only a very low dosage of Klonopin, which he hopes to taper off over the next few weeks.

After years of hell, Henry is now free of depression, and is confident socially and in his work. Aside from these enormous benefits, he is delighted at his greatly improved sexual enjoyment and functioning. Although a man of science who recognizes that the herb must be working on a variety of brain chemicals, Henry regards the changes brought about by St. John's wort as nothing less than a miracle.

Jake: A Struggling Screenwriter

Jake is a twenty-nine-year-old freelance writer and health food store owner who is currently trying to write and sell screenplays. He has suffered from feelings of sadness, fatigue, and anxiety off and on since the age of three, when his parents were divorced. He remembers being sick a lot as a child and getting into many fights at school. He was the class clown and was often in trouble with teachers.

Jake's depressions went undiagnosed until age twenty-two, when he felt extremely sad and dejected. He had recently completed college and didn't know what he wanted to do with his life. He was working as a fund-raiser for disadvantaged children, but was tired much of the time and had a hard time performing his tasks. When he consulted me in the fall, he had quit work and was home sleeping most of the time.

Jake had previously been treated with Prozac, but it didn't help his lack of energy, which was one of his main symptoms, and made him feel spacey. I then treated him with Wellbutrin in high dosages. Although the drug made him feel more energetic and less down in the dumps, it also made him angry and irritable and he developed a nasty edge in his dealings with other people that was quite uncharacteristic for him. To combat these unwelcome effects of Wellbutrin, I added a second mood-regulating drug, lithium carbonate. In addition, he also received psychotherapy and light therapy. This combination of treatments was quite effective, and by the end of the year, he had enough energy to acquire two part-time jobs and felt about as good as he could recall. He was bothered, however, by medication side effects, such as sleep disturbance and continued aggressive feelings despite the placating effects of lithium.

After several years on this combination, Jake stopped his medications because he wanted to see how he would do without them. He felt fine until he moved to a new city with his girlfriend. He had always had difficulties with transitions and he felt the old, familiar fatigue and anxiety coming back to him. He consulted an internist, who restarted him on Wellbutrin.

Once again, he began to feel unpleasantly edgy. At Jake's request, the internist prescribed a different antidepressant, Zoloft, which helped his mood somewhat but decreased his sex drive a great deal. Not only was he less interested in sex, but he also had difficulty with erections and orgasms. He began to avoid sex because it was uncomfortable for him not to be able to perform, and it affected his self-esteem.

Jake read about St. John's wort in the popular press and, coincidentally, I had just begun to treat his mother with the herbal extract with excellent results. Since he is interested in alternative medicines, he put himself on St. John's wort, 300 mg three times a day, and gradually phased out the Zoloft. His sex drive, mood, and energy level improved markedly following the introduction of St. John's wort. The only side effect was mild indigestion, which responded readily to antacids and was short-lived.

Jake's mood and energy levels are as good as they have ever been and he finally feels "like a normal person." He is grateful to the herbal remedy for helping him so much, even though he recognizes that he has also worked very hard to feel better about himself and his life. This work has involved therapy and self-reflection, regular exercise, and actively avoiding toxic influences and negative attitudes. He plans to move to Los Angeles, where he is more likely to succeed as a screenwriter, and feels optimistic even though his chosen course is a difficult and risky one, and even though he has recently broken up with a girlfriend to whom he was deeply attached.

Although Jake shifted successfully from Zoloft to St. John's wort on his own, I recommend that if you are contemplating making such a switch you do so under a doctor's supervision, in case side effects develop that would benefit from medical attention. But Jake had clearly learned some of the key principles of antidepressant management during his years of psychiatric care and did a good job of juggling his own medications. He recalled, for example, that if at all possible you should try not to stop an antidepressant abruptly. To do so is to court withdrawal side effects such as dizziness, sleep disruption, and flu-like symptoms, to name just a few. Also, sudden withdrawal can result in a rapid decline back into depression again. So Jake was wise to taper his Zoloft gradually.

Jake recognized that finding the right antidepressant is only one aspect of the treatment of depression. I discuss how to incorporate St. John's wort into an antidepressant lifestyle in a later chapter (see chapter 11). Jake's move to Los Angeles also promises to be a healthy choice for him, as it is more likely to offer him the career opportunities he needs in order to feel professionally fulfilled.

Brent: A Litigator Who Needed His Edge

Brent, a highly successful litigator, suffered from mild but nagging symptoms of anxiety and difficulty enjoying life. I treated his symptoms effectively with Zoloft, but it reduced his sex drive and ability to enjoy sex to an unacceptable degree. In addition, it made him excessively bland and he felt that it caused him to lose the fighting edge necessary for a successful litigator. I switched him to Wellbutrin, which once again treated his symptoms effectively, but now he was excessively irritable and lacked the measure of calm control needed for successful negotiations. An uneasy balance was struck by combining these two drugs, increasing the one and decreasing the other according to the way he felt and the varying demands of his work. Switching from the combination of synthetic antidepressants to 900 mg a day of St. John's wort proved to be a completely satisfactory solution, successfully treating his depressive symptoms without causing sexual or behavioral side effects. He felt calmer and less anxious without losing his edge.

Emily: Fed Up with Side Effects

Emily originally came to me because life seemed to have lost its sparkle for her. She had always enjoyed social and cultural events, but in the months preceding our first visit, she had lost her zest for even the most scintillating company and the best art exhibitions that the major galleries in Washington, D.C., have to offer. Wellbutrin restored her interest in her life, but at a cost—dry mouth and eyes. Eventually these side effects became intolerable and some alternative approach was clearly needed. Once again, a switch to St. John's wort, 900 mg per day, took care of her depressive symptoms without causing any side effects at all.

Henry, Jake, Brent, and Emily are among the relatively fortunate individuals whose symptoms were reversed by St. John's wort alone. For many people, however, this is not possible and they end up on combinations of St. John's wort and synthetic antidepressants. The good news is that these combinations are often highly effective and often lack the side effects that would result if the synthetic antidepressant were used in the higher dosages that would be necessary without the assistance of St. John's wort. In addition, if such combinations are properly supervised and monitored, they are generally quite safe. Here are some examples of people who did well on such combinations.

Vanessa, A Retiring Scientist: Adding an SSRI to St. John's Wort

Vanessa is a scientist in her mid-forties who has suffered from recurrent depressions for as long as she can remember. During her depressed periods, which can last for months, Vanessa withdraws from others, needs to sleep a great deal of the time, has difficulty concentrating, and feels sad and worthless. Although a highly intelligent woman, she lacks confidence in her abilities and for many years has worked in a job that is beneath her skills and qualifications. She was reluctant to ask her boss for a promotion, however, as she questioned whether she deserved it and feared that her request would be denied, which would confirm her sense of worthlessness.

In the past, Vanessa was treated with Zoloft during the worst parts of her depressions, requiring dosages of as much as 150 mg per day in order to obtain therapeutic effects. Although the medication removed the most painful aspects of her depressions, it sedated her. In addition, she felt that it took away her range of feelings, making her unable to respond fully to the events in her life, unable to muster much joy in response to good news or feel appropriately sad when bad things happened. As she described it, "I felt zombified," and for this reason she would discontinue the medication shortly after emerging from her depression.

Vanessa happened to be in one of her depressions when St. John's wort was becoming widely publicized in the United States and she decided to try the herbal remedy at the usual dosage of 300 mg three times a day. After a few weeks, she felt it was helping her, but now, instead of her feelings being flattened out, she felt greater swings in mood than before. Within the same day, her mood would fluctuate several times, from good humor to despair and discouragement. On the advice of a psychiatrist, Vanessa added Zoloft to the mix, trying only 50 mg per day, one third of the amount that she had previously required. For the first time in her life, she felt good in a sustained way without feeling medicated. As she put it, "I feel like myself at my best all of the time. I get upset when things go wrong and happy when they go right, but they feel like normal feelings, not depression or like being a dull zombie."

Since feeling better, Vanessa has managed to travel and socialize much more freely and happily than had ever previously been possible. She also plucked up the courage to ask her boss for a promotion, which he readily agreed she deserved and promptly took the necessary steps to make it happen.

For another patient of mine, a combination of Prozac and St. John's wort also appears promising. The young woman in question wanted to switch from 20 mg a day of Prozac to St. John's wort because she had gained weight while on Prozac. Several weeks after the switch she began to feel depressed and we decided to restart her Prozac at a lower dosage of 10 mg a day in conjunction with the St. John's wort. This combination appeared to hold her depressive symptoms in check, but we have yet to see whether it helps her lose the weight she gained on the higher dose of Prozac.

The lesson to be learned from this young woman and from Vanessa is that one does not have to choose between herbal and pharmaceutical antidepressants. The best outcome may come from mixing the two. I would not, however, recommend trying such mixtures on your own, since medications can interact adversely as well as favorably and one is best off having a doctor involved to minimize the chance of that happening.

Adding St. John's Wort to Current Antidepressant Medications

If one treats a large number of depressed patients, as I do, the use of antidepressant combinations is standard operating procedure as the antidepressants frequently don't work completely when administered individually. If one has to be depressed, the late twentieth century is not such a bad time for it, as there is an ever-increasing array of available medications that act on different elements of the neurons responsible for transmitting the signals that regulate our moods. The skillful clinician, working in collaboration with an observant patient, can mix and blend these medications in such a way as to maximize their benefits while minimizing their side effects.

St. John's wort appears to work very well in combination with all antidepressants except for the MAOIs, such as Parnate or Nardil, where adding them can be dangerous. Combining MAOIs with other antidepressants has been reported to result in serious overheating of the body and disruption of brain functioning, which, in severe cases, can prove fatal. Even though it is reasonably safe to mix St. John's wort with antidepressants other than MAOIs, this is not to say that these medications should be mindlessly shaken into a cocktail in their full dosage. After all, if these medications can interact with one another in positive ways that enhance their antidepressant effects, they also have the potential to enhance one another's side effects. When mixing medications, it is important therefore to move more cautiously with dosages and timing. See page 183 for further information on combining St. John's wort and antidepressants.

In certain instances I have seen people maintain their antidepressant response despite decreasing the dosage of antidepressants that were giving them unpleasant side effects by adding St. John's wort. For example, Fred, a fifty-two-year-old computer scientist, wrote to tell me that he was able to decrease the dosage of his antidepressant (Wellbutrin) by adding St. John's wort to his medication regimen. According to Fred, the addition of St. John's wort "takes the edge off feelings of anxiety and depression and flips the switch from negative to positive." As he put it, "I feel like good things will happen—a feeling that I am okay, not perfect, but me. I sense that life is going to get better."

I have similarly observed in my own patients the highly beneficial interactions between St. John's wort and other antidepressants, sometimes subtle, sometimes very robust. In rare instances, however, people can develop side effects on such combinations, such as high blood pressure, feelings of being "wired" or "hyper," confusion, or restlessness. If any of these symptoms develop, report them to your doctor without delay.

Many of my patients are on complicated combinations of antidepressants and I have been pleasantly surprised to find that the addition of St. John's wort may nevertheless provide additional antidepressant protection even in people with depressions that have been hard to reverse. Sometimes the addition of the herb has been so helpful that it has been possible to decrease the dose of some of the other medications or even to remove one or more of them, thereby simplifying the overall medication regimen. As always, the key to successfully combining medications—and St. John's wort is no exception in this regard—is to change dosages slowly and observe carefully for any untoward effects.

Remember: If you are on an MAOI such as Parnate or Nardil, do not take St. John's wort. Also, if you have discontinued an MAOI, wait at least two weeks before starting St. John's wort.

Combining St. John's Wort with Stimulant Medications

There has been a resurgence in the use of stimulant medications, such as Ritalin and Dexedrine, with the increased awareness and recognition of the problem of adult attention deficit disorder (ADD). Since it is not uncommon to find both depression and ADD in the same person, the question will arise as to the safety of combining stimulants with the herbal antidepressant. At this time there appears to be no reason to avoid doing so provided, once again, that it is done under a doctor's supervision, using the usual rules of starting low and going slow, as the following two case studies will indicate.

Dick, an economist in his early fifties, was referred to a sleep clinic by his wife, who suspected him of having sleep apnea because of his snoring. After sleep studies were performed, sleep apnea was ruled out, and instead he was diagnosed as suffering from narcolepsy, a condition characterized by waking during the night and severe drowsiness during the day. The drowsiness can reach dangerous levels, as patients may doze off at the wheel of a car or fall asleep at other inopportune times. Other curious features of this disorder are a tendency to have hallucinations just as one is falling asleep and to lose muscle tone and collapse while awake, often as part of an emotional response such as laughing. It has been suggested that the dormouse in *Alice in Wonderland* might have been suffering from narcolepsy, as he was always falling asleep and collapsing into the teapot.

Dick's symptoms of narcolepsy were effectively treated with the stimulant Ritalin, but after his drowsiness cleared, he realized that he was left with aspects of his personality that displeased him, particularly shyness and excessive cautiousness. He would hesitate to initiate conversations, to offer his opinions in group meetings, or to assert himself in the workplace. In addition, he continued to overeat and gain weight and his sleep disturbances persisted to some degree. Even though he was not actually depressed and was able to experience pleasure in aspects of his life, his psychiatrist thought he might be suffering from a type of depression and prescribed St. John's wort, 900 mg per day.

The very day after starting the herb, he felt buoyant, which was very surprising to him, as he had read that it takes weeks for the herb to exert its effects. He knew that something unusual was going on because although he had bicycled into work every day for months, he had never before initiated a conversation with one of his fellow bikers. That day he did—and he has been less shy ever since, less self-effacing and more inclined to speak up. Even confrontations, which he would assiduously avoid in the past, now no longer seem so daunting. He is contributing more in meetings and feels more engaged. Others have noted these changes even more than he has and have pointed them out to him. His psychiatrist has pushed the dosage of St. John's wort higher—to 1,250 mg per day—in an attempt to get the maximum benefit from it. Best of all, he has not noticed any side effects whatsoever.

I had occasion to combine St. John's wort and stimulants in treating Zack, a seventeen-year-old boy with a history of both long-standing depression and ADD. When he first came to see me, he was on one of the older antidepressants, nortriptyline. Even though he was on a relatively low dosage of the antidepressant, he noted a distinct decrease in his interest in girls after starting the medication. "I am still interested in them up here," he remarked, pointing in the vicinity of his brain, "but it doesn't seem to be connected with down there," he said, his finger drifting downward. This was clearly a case for St. John's wort. In my usual fashion, I gradually added the herbal antidepressant while tapering the conventional antidepressant. On St. John's wort alone, Zack felt too giddy, impulsive, and unconstrained, so I reduced the dosage of St. John's wort and reintroduced the nortriptyline at an even lower dosage than before. He declared the mix to be perfect. He no longer felt depressed, was no longer impulsive, and experienced a welcome return of his interest in girls, both emotionally and physically.

Now it was time for Zack to go off to college, and concentration and focus became major problems for him, as they invariably are for people with ADD. I introduced the stimulant Dexedrine, 5 mg twice a day, to the mix, which helped him with his attention and his studies. He reported no problematic side effects from the combination and is now enjoying school, both socially and intellectually.

———

In summary, St. John's wort can frequently be used instead of conventional antidepressants and some patients currently being treated with synthetic antidepressants may benefit from switching to the herbal remedy. Such switches should not be made without good reason, however, but only if the response to current treatment is inadequate or if side effects are unacceptable. Always involve your doctor when you want to switch or combine medications. In those for whom St. John's wort alone is inadequate, combining the herb with other antidepressants often results in a satisfying combination that is both effective and well tolerated.

6

BEATING THE WINTER BLUES WITH ST. JOHN'S WORT AND LIGHT

Every November, as the days became shorter and daylight began to fade, Sarah, now in her early fifties, would feel an old, familiar affliction come over her. An artist, she sees the world in colors. Autumn was a gray season. She would have difficulty waking up in the morning and would sense her energy ebbing away. Although normally a competent person, even simple tasks would now feel impossible, and she had lost the joy of living. One of her few pleasures was eating—comfort foods such as grilled cheese sandwiches, scones, or buttered toast. She would gain five to ten pounds every winter that she would lose again the following summer.

Her depression would deepen in December, made worse by memories of a child she had lost in that month many years before and the departure of her children, who would spend time with her ex-husband during that season. The approach of the holidays compounded her misery, making her anxious that she would not be able to celebrate Christmas properly with her children. At times she was unable to get her Christmas cards out and make all the necessary preparations for the holidays, which would leave her feeling guilty and inadequate as a mother and despairing that things would ever turn out as she wanted them to. She would become reclusive and not want to venture out at all. When she did go out, she would hide in a corner and if someone spoke to her, would nod her head but not really participate. The world would look completely black to her then and sometimes suicide would beckon to her as a welcome relief from her pain.

Things would improve in January, which was lighter and brighter, in part because of the sunlight reflected off the snow, and she found it easier to get through the days. February, on the other hand, was dark once again and she would only begin to emerge from her depression in a solid and predictable way when March arrived. For the rest of the year she was fine.

Sarah first saw a psychiatrist for treatment of her depression when she was in her twenties. A major factor contributing to her difficulties was the death of her father when she was thirteen and unresolved feelings around that. Later troubles included the death of a child when Sarah was thirty-one years old and a "horrendous" divorce. Despite psychotherapy being helpful, her cyclical depressions persisted and she was given antidepressant medications to deal with them. Unfortunately, she was unable to handle any of the synthetic antidepressants that were tried. Prozac and other medications caused her heart to beat rapidly and did not feel right for her body. She had always been very sensitive to medications of all kinds; even Excedrin made her feel "high," spacey and giddy.

One type of treatment that helped her a great deal, without any side effects, was light therapy. She obtained a special light box and would begin to use it starting at the end of October. She would sit in front of the lights twice a day, for half an hour in the morning while eating breakfast and half an hour in the evening at dinnertime. The first year she used the lights she managed to get her Christmas cards out on time and was actually able to plan a New Year's party. But even though the lights prevented her from hitting the bottom of her depression, she still felt low and the world still looked dark and gray.

About eighteen months ago Sarah, who describes herself as "an old sixties kid, an Adele Davis kind of person," heard about St. John's wort, which appealed to her because of its herbal nature. She began using 300 mg twice a day during one of her depressions. Almost immediately she noted an evening out of her moods and enjoyed not being whipsawed by her customary highs and lows. For the sake of convenience, she changed her dosing schedule to 600 mg in the morning and found that that worked equally well. Now she is able to deal with her problems and be in a stable and upbeat mood, free of depression all year round. She sings the praises of St. John's wort to "all kinds of people."

St. John's wort clearly helped Sara's winter depressions enormously and she is now able to get her cards out early and look forward to the season. Christmastime, which was formerly so very difficult for her, now no longer seems grim. Even though she continues to use light therapy during the gray days of winter, the addition of St. John's wort has made a critical difference in her ability to feel happy and functional throughout this black season.

Seasonal Affective Disorder (SAD)

Sarah suffers from a typical case of seasonal affective disorder, or SAD. People with this condition are very sensitive to the amounts of light in their environment and become depressed when these levels fall below a certain threshold, such as during the short, dark days of winter. Although this problem probably has a genetic basis, the severity of winter depressions depends on the amount of light in the environment of a susceptible person. Often, people with SAD who have lived in different locations report that their problem was worse the farther away they lived from the equator, with depressions lasting longer and being more severe than when they lived in more tropical climes. For some reason not yet understood, women are more susceptible than men to SAD, especially when they are in their reproductive years.

When depressed, people with SAD tend to oversleep. Often, they just feel like curling up in bed and being left alone. They empathize with hibernating bears who are free to laze away the winter without the responsibilities that beset us humans all year round. Such responsibilities often overwhelm the person with winter depression, who can barely rouse herself and get going, let alone tackle the chores, work, and personal commitments that are part of ordinary living. As a result, the person with SAD often feels like a failure, and anxiety and depression are always close at hand. One source of comfort is food, especially sweets and starches, which are consumed in great amounts, resulting in unwelcome weight gain.

Seasonal affective disorder is extremely common and has been estimated to affect about 6 percent of adults in the United States. Another 14 percent are estimated to suffer from a milder form of the condition, subsyndromal SAD, or the winter blues. Although most people with the milder version of SAD do not seek out medical attention, the dark, short, winter days nevertheless interfere with their productivity and creativity and make life feel dreary and dull. It is estimated that approximately one in five people in the United States suffers from emotional or behavioral disturbances as a result of winter.

Light deprivation, for any reason, will tend to depress these susceptible individuals. Two or three cloudy days in a row, a windowless office, or a basement apartment are all quite likely to lead to a lack of energy and a slump in mood. Once the connection is made between the amount of environmental light and mood, however, the condition feels immediately less burdensome. As Sarah put it, "Understanding the problem is half the battle." The other half of the battle can be won with the help of light therapy, St. John's wort, and other antidepressant strategies.

Standard Treatments for SAD

Light therapy has been the primary treatment for the symptoms of winter depression. Patients with SAD typically sit in front of a light fixture, which emits light about twenty times as bright as ordinary room light, for a varying amount of time each day. Treatments usually need to be repeated on a daily basis throughout the autumn and winter.

Another way of bringing more light into the bedroom is to use a dawn simulator, an electronic device that attaches to a bedside lamp and can be programmed to turn the lamp on gradually at a preset time of day, thereby simulating some of the features of a summer dawn.

Even though both light boxes and dawn simulators have been found to be effective in treating patients with seasonal affective disorder, many patients do not respond fully to these treatments. Antidepressant medications have frequently been prescribed for such incomplete responders. As St. John's wort appears to be effective in reversing the symptoms of SAD, affected individuals now have an alternative treatment option.

Using St. John's Wort in SAD

Interestingly, the earliest systematic twentieth-century study of the effects of St. John's wort on depression was inspired by the observation that hypericum is a light-sensitive substance and that rats given hypericum and then placed in bright light appeared to become more active. To date there is only one study on the use of St. John's wort in SAD patients. In this 1994 study, "Hypericum in the Treatment of Seasonal Affective Disorders," Dr. Siegfried Kasper and colleagues compared two groups of ten SAD patients, one exposed to bright light in the morning for two hours a day for four weeks and one to much dimmer light for the same amount of time. Both groups received St. John's wort, 900 mg per day, and both groups responded very well over the four-week trial. Given the way in which the study was designed, it is difficult to draw definite conclusions from it. Because there was no placebo group, the evidence for a specific effect for St. John's wort was not completely clear-cut. Since both groups did equally well, there is a temptation to conclude that the addition of bright light does not enhance the antidepressant effects of St. John's wort in SAD.

Nevertheless, both groups responded extremely well, and had there been a placebo group, I wager that it would not have fared as well as those on St. John's wort. Even though the relatively small number of subjects does not enable us to comment with any confidence on the potential benefit of adding light therapy to St. John's wort, in my experience with treating hundreds of SAD patients, light therapy and antidepressants almost always work well together. The light therapy enhances the effects of the antidepressant and the antidepressant cuts down on the amount of time needed in front of the lights. There is no reason to suppose that the same beneficial interaction will not occur when it comes to the use of St. John's wort. In my opinion, Sarah's happy experience in using these two treatments in conjunction with each other will prove to be the norm. Most patients with SAD suffer only mild to moderate depressions—the very type that have been shown to respond well to St. John's wort.

There are different ways in which light therapy and St. John's wort could be combined. You could reason that since light therapy is the more established of the two treatments for SAD, it would make sense to begin to use light treatment as you enter the usual season of risk. As soon as it feels as though the light therapy is not fully doing the job, you could then add St. John's wort in the same dosing regimen outlined elsewhere in this book. Another approach would be to start with St. John's wort and add light therapy only if it is necessary.

Although Dr. Kasper's group found no harmful effects to the eye after treating patients with four weeks of light therapy in conjunction with St. John's wort, there is a theoretical concern that over the long haul the light-sensitizing effects of the herbal antidepressant may produce harmful effects on the eyes. Since such speculations by definition involve watching people over long periods, it will not be possible to address them definitively for years. Even so, it is good to be aware of this possible interaction and to use less light if you are also taking St. John's wort than you would if light were the only antidepressant treatment you were receiving. This should be easily managed, as you will be benefiting from two remedies rather than just one. In addition, people have a natural inclination to use as little light therapy as is needed to obtain an antidepressant response.

One tip worth bearing in mind whenever you use an antidepressant to treat SAD or the winter blues is that the dosage needed usually varies with the season. For example, 300–600 mg of St. John's wort might be sufficient in the autumn and spring, but larger doses may be necessary to combat the more severe symptoms that may occur in the depths of winter.

How Long Should You Continue to Treat Your Winter Depression?

In general, those who recover spontaneously from their winter depressions during the summer months are able to stop their antidepressant treatments—be they light or medications—when long, sunny days arrive. The same principle should apply to St. John's wort, and I would recommend that those who normally feel fine in the summer discontinue the herbal antidepressant at that time. On the other hand, those who feel somewhat depressed all the time, but more so in the winter, are likely to benefit from St. John's wort all year round. These people might require dosage adjustments, with more St. John's wort needed in the winter and less in the summer.

For further information about the effects of the seasons on mood and behavior, and strategies to deal with the difficulties caused by the short, dark days of winter or other forms of light deprivation, I refer the interested reader to my book *Winter Blues* (Guilford Books, 1998), which deals with these topics in greater detail.

7

ST. JOHN'S WORT IN THE ELDERLY

*Antidepressant effects of hypericum have been con-
firmed in several clinical studies that have compared
this compound to placebo as well as to standard antidepressants. . . . One of the most important features is
that side effects occur rarely. This benign side effect profile may make hypericum a particularly attractive
choice for treating mild-to-moderate depression in our
elderly patients.*

—MICHAEL JENIKE, M.D., *JOURNAL OF
GERIATRIC PSYCHIATRY AND NEUROLOGY,* 1994

One result of the success of modern medicine in conquering
the diseases of childhood and middle life is the aging of
our population and the progressive increase in those of us who
can be regarded as elderly, regardless of how we define that
term. Depression is very common among the elderly, and its
more serious form, major depression, has been estimated to
affect approximately one in seven individuals over age sixty-
five in community settings and as many as one in four individuals in nursing homes. An index of the severity of this problem
is the fact that the highest suicide rates occur among our
elderly citizens. The elderly have many reasons to be depressed,
including physical ailments, isolation from family, the loss of
friends, and financial difficulties, to name just a few. This leads
to the common misconception even among health care workers
that depression may be a natural and justifiable response to an
elderly person's life circumstances. Nevertheless, regardless of
how adverse a person's life circumstances may be, wherever

depression is encountered, including among the elderly, it is certainly worth treating. This will often result in a markedly improved quality of life even though it will not necessarily change the realistic basis for a person's sorrows.

Because St. John's wort has only recently come to the attention of clinicians in the United States, our doctors have very little experience with its use in older patients with depression. Yet, as Dr. Michael Jenike points out in the editorial quoted above, St. John's wort would seem like a very reasonable antidepressant for those elderly people who are depressed. As our population ages, medications that are suited to older people will surely become increasingly important, and considering the widespread prevalence of depression in the elderly, it is a particular blessing that nature's own apothecary, in the form of St. John's wort, appears to have yielded so excellent a remedy for this group of people.

Perhaps the person with the most experience in treating elderly patients, with St. John's wort is Dr. Hans-Peter Volz, professor of psychiatry at the University of Jena, formerly in East Germany. He estimates that he has treated approximately seventy depressed patients over age sixty-five with St. John's wort in dosages of up to 900 mg per day. He is comfortable with recommending it as a first-line treatment in mildly depressed elderly patients, though he is still inclined to use conventional antidepressants for those who are moderately or severely depressed. He acknowledges, however, that his practice of not using St. John's wort as a first-line treatment in more seriously depressed cases is not based on his direct experience that it is not of benefit for such people but rather on the absence of sufficient controlled study data on the use of St. John's wort in severe depression.

Dr. Volz reports excellent antidepressant effects, with very few side effects, in the elderly people he has treated. In addition, he has noted no adverse interactions between St. John's wort and the many drugs that elderly people often need to take for ailments accumulated over a lifetime. He emphasizes the need to wait six to eight weeks before passing judgment as to whether the herbal remedy is working or not. Here are two cases from Dr. Volz's clinical files.

Greta: No "Chemical Stuff," but Herbs Are Not Dangerous

When Greta, a sixty-nine-year-old woman referred to Dr. Volz by her general practitioner, was asked what was troubling her, depression was the furthest condition from her mind. Instead, she complained of many physical ailments—headache, stomachache, tiredness, and an unpleasant taste in her mouth. Her general practitioner was unable to find any physical explanation for these symptoms and the only abnormality he could detect was a slight problem with cardiac conduction, as measured by an EKG. She had complained of sleep difficulties, for which she had been treated with sleeping pills with some success.

When Dr. Volz questioned her, it became apparent that her difficulties had begun about two years before, shortly after her husband had died unexpectedly of a heart attack. Despite having enough money and a close relationship with her son, who lived in the same town and would visit her twice a week, Greta complained of sadness and hopelessness but, she hastened to add, "only when I am alone." Dr. Volz tried to explain to her that her symptoms might be due to depression, but she vehemently objected to such an explanation. When he suggested that she might benefit from a drug such as Prozac, she refused to take any synthetic antidepressants, insisting "that's all chemical stuff." After two further visits with Dr. Volz, he suggested that she try St. John's wort. To his astonishment, she immediately agreed to take this because "herbs are not dangerous."

Dr. Volz started Greta on St. John's wort, 900 mg per day. He noticed no improvement until she had been on the herbal remedy for six weeks, and it took another ten weeks before Greta's symptoms were reduced to a significant degree. Greta remains convinced that the improvement she has enjoyed on St. John's wort does not mean that she suffered from depression for which treatment would have been required. Instead, she attributes her improved mood to "nonspecific" effects of the herb. Dr. Volz sees no need to challenge that belief. She is no longer depressed and her mood has been stable without any adverse effects whatsoever. That is reward enough for a caring doctor.

Anna: Success Where Other Medications Had Failed

Anna was seventy-eight when she was first referred to Dr. Volz by a local internist. By that age, her experiences with recurrent episodes of depression went back a quarter of a century. In the early 1980s she was treated with lithium carbonate, which was discontinued when it resulted in thyroid troubles. In the early 1990s she was treated with amitriptyline, one of the older antidepressants, which caused her to have severe dry mouth and, on one occasion, an episode of fainting when she got up one night to go to the toilet. Then Prozac, 20 mg a day, was tried, and even though it helped her depression to some degree, it caused unbearable sleep problems. Sometimes it would take her as long as two hours to fall asleep at night and then she would wake an average of three times during the course of the night.

When Anna consulted Dr. Volz, he judged her to be moderately depressed while on Prozac, scoring twenty-one points, a high score on the well-known Hamilton Depression Rating Scale, on which the higher the score, the more depressed the individual. A score of twenty-one suggests a moderately severe depression. Because of the profound sleep difficulties on Prozac, Dr. Volz decided to switch Anna to St. John's wort. He did this without any overlap between medications, immediately discontinuing her Prozac and starting St. John's wort at 900 mg per day. Four days later Anna reported an improvement in the quality of her sleep, but her mood had deteriorated slightly and she now scored twenty-four on the Hamilton Rating Scale. Her dosage of St. John's wort was increased to 1,800 mg per day, and after three weeks her rating score dropped to twenty, after six weeks to fifteen, and after another four weeks to ten. Anna's depression continues to improve. Once again, St. John's wort triumphed where other medications had failed.

There are several lessons to be learned from Dr. Volz and his patients. For many people like Greta, herbal remedies are simply more acceptable than synthetic drugs. Perhaps it is because we are used to eating fruits and vegetables that swallowing plant extracts feels more natural to us than swallowing synthetic medicines. Even though we need properly conducted studies to definitively declare an antidepressant to be effective, it is hard not to become a believer in the antidepressant effects of St. John's wort when one encounters patients such as Greta. Adamantly opposed to the very idea that she was depressed, and uninformed about the purported antidepressant effects of St. John's wort, her symptoms nevertheless responded completely to the herbal remedy. Because St. John's wort does not appear to have any adverse effect on electrical conduction in the heart, Dr. Volz felt quite comfortable using it to treat Greta's depression even though her EKG had revealed some abnormalities in her cardiac conduction.

In Anna's case, we see the importance of persevering with an antidepressant treatment. After she was switched from Prozac to St. John's wort, she initially appeared to get worse before her slow but progressive improvement over the course of the next several months. Such a transient decline in mood is not uncommon when antidepressants are being switched and adjusted, and it is no reason to be discouraged with the new line of treatment. Dr. Volz correctly persevered with his game plan. On the other hand, if a decline persists for weeks, it should be regarded as a reason to reevaluate the treatment strategy and consider an alternative antidepressant.

Anna's depression was moderately severe when she first consulted Dr. Volz and had apparently been somewhat worse before she started Prozac. Nevertheless, St. John's wort successfully turned her depression around, indicating once again the potency of the herbal remedy. Despite this potency, the mildness of the herbal antidepressant was apparent in the ease with which this elderly woman was able to tolerate it in dosages that are twice as high as those widely recommended for the treatment of mild to moderate depression. This was in marked contrast to the synthetic antidepressants she had previously taken and on which she had developed unacceptable side effects. It is quite likely that the customary dosage of 900 mg per day of St. John's wort will prove to be insufficient for some individuals who might safely be able to tolerate higher dosages. It would be beneficial to explore more fully the desirable dosage range for the use of the herbal antidepressant.

There is only one point of practice on which I differ from Dr. Volz, which is that I generally recommend tapering any antidepressant before switching to another one rather than stopping it suddenly. In my experience, stopping an antidepressant suddenly is more likely to result in withdrawal symptoms, such as sleep difficulties or irritability, as compared with tapering it more gradually.

St. John's Wort and the Elderly in Germany: A Part of General Practice

In Germany the use of St. John's wort for elderly depressed people is by no means confined to specialists such as Dr. Volz. Rather, it is part of ordinary clinical practice and is prescribed by general practitioners. As part of my attempt to get a picture of the usage patterns of St. John's wort in Germany, I distributed my survey questionnaires to pharmacies there and received several replies from elderly users of the herb. My colleague, Dr. Alexander Neumeister, a psychiatrist in Vienna, interviewed some of these respondents. Here are three of their stories.

Elsa, a sixty-five-year-old retired nurse, always regarded herself as an anxious and sorrowful person, never as happy as others. She had been treated on and off with the early antidepressants, but stopped them after a few days because she could not tolerate their side effects. After her retirement she became markedly depressed and a general practitioner urged her to take St. John's wort. Although she was convinced it would not work, she agreed to do so because it was an herbal extract. Within two weeks of starting the herbal antidepressant (900 mg per day), she felt her anxiety and depression lift and is now able to enjoy her life and spends time taking care of her grandchildren and going on vacations. She has observed no side effects.

Irene, an eighty-year-old retired schoolteacher, had never suffered depression until three years ago, when she developed heart problems. She had several heart attacks and suffered from the pain of angina when she exercised. She was on medications for high blood pressure. Hospitalized for these problems, she was extremely fearful but regarded these fears as excessive because, as she put it, her life was not at immediate risk and others in the hospital were more seriously ill than she was. She had difficulty falling asleep and staying asleep through the night, and stopped socializing with friends even though she had previously been a gregarious person. Her doctor prescribed St. John's wort, starting with 300 mg at night. At this low dosage it did not help her, but when he increased the dosage to 900 mg per day, her sleep pattern improved, her depression lifted, and she no longer felt anxious. At about the same time, she began to feel better physically. She has remained on St. John's wort for three years without suffering any relapse of her depressive symptoms.

Gerda, a seventy-two-year-old housewife, describes herself as a very nervous person with many physical symptoms, especially abdominal pains after eating, for which she has taken medications over the years. She has observed a seasonal pattern to her physical and emotional problems, which are worse during the winter. Six months ago she began to feel so depressed, anxious, and irritable that her children took her to a psychiatrist. He initially prescribed Paxil, but she developed feelings of nausea, became more anxious and agitated, and stopped the medication after two weeks. On St. John's wort, 900 mg per day, her anxiety has settled down and her abdominal pains have almost disappeared. In addition, she no longer has a need for daily pain medications.

There is no reason to believe that St. John's wort will not prove as effective and well tolerated in elderly individuals on this side of the Atlantic as it has in Germany. Even though relatively few older people have taken the herb for depression in this country, here are a few reports that have come to my attention. By now there must certainly be many more such success stories.

Gabrielle: Rediscovering Hope

Gabrielle, at age sixty-two, has had many roles during her life: wife to a foreign diplomat, mother of five, indefatigable fundraiser for her favorite charities, and formerly a public relations consultant for the fashion industry. But none of these roles prepared her for the role that many of us dread and for which none of us is truly prepared when the shock hits us, namely, the role of cancer patient.

In retrospect, warning signs had extended back for many months but, as is often the case, they were missed by both Gabrielle and her physicians. She had previously suffered from colitis, so the typical bowel symptoms of cancer were easily explained away. But after her symptoms had continued for five months, she underwent a colonoscopy and a large tumor of the colon was diagnosed. This was removed surgically but, unfortunately, the cancer had already spread to the liver by that time.

Gabrielle had never previously been depressed even though depression runs in her family. Her mother had been affected by the condition, as had three of her four sisters, two of whom had lengthy stays in psychiatric hospitals and one of whom committed suicide. After the surgery, Gabrielle could understand how this third sister had been driven to such a desperate act, as she herself was overcome by a "tremendous" depression. She felt sad and tearful much of the time. Riddled with guilt, she blamed herself for not having attended to the symptoms of her tumor more promptly. She couldn't eat and wanted to throw up. Normally a very sociable person, she didn't want to talk to anyone or answer the phone. Gabrielle spent much of the day lying in bed, looking at the ceiling. Her legs were heavy and she was unable to walk, which was perhaps just as well because she had thoughts of running into the street in front of the oncoming traffic and putting an end to it all.

Her doctor prescribed Zoloft, which she took for three days but stopped because it suppressed her appetite, made her feel nauseated, and interfered with her sleep. Another antidepressant was prescribed but she was reluctant to take it as it came with warnings against going into the sun and she and her family were on the verge of taking a trip to Puerto Rico to see one of her children. In Puerto Rico Gabrielle's husband told her about St. John's wort and there seemed to be little harm in trying the herbal remedy. Even though the setting was lovely and she was with family, she still felt very down, "like a drag on everybody."

Gabrielle bought some St. John's wort in a health food store in Puerto Rico and began by taking one capsule twice a day. It worked "like magic," and after a week she felt wonderful. She has been on it now for two months and all symptoms of depression have left even though she needs to go for chemotherapy once a week. "I go out, I talk to people again, and I don't think of my physical illness." Gabrielle attributes some of her recovery to the loving support of her family and vacations they have taken together, but she is sure that none of this would have been possible without the help of St. John's wort, which, to her relief, has been without any side effects whatsoever. So excited is she about the herb that she suggested that her daughter, who was also depressed, start St. John's wort at the same time she did. According to Gabrielle, "My daughter is very happy with its effects." Gabrielle has been told that the prognosis for her cancer is good, and she is determined to live her life as fully as possible rather than "with one leg here and one leg there." Now that her depression is better, she is able to make good on this resolution.

Frieda: A "Gay Depressed" Pianist

If Gabrielle is convinced that St. John's wort has helped her depression, for Frieda, a seventy-seven-year-old concert pianist, the jury is still out on the matter. Her psychiatrist, Dr. Thomas Wehr, is more certain that it has helped with the quality of her sleep at night and her subsequent wakefulness during the day.

Born in Hungary, Frieda was a child prodigy who learned to play the piano at age two and a half, while still in diapers. Seventy-five years later she is still playing the piano, currently in an upscale department store where she is so popular that families have written to the store management telling them what a treasure they have in her. Not only does she play standard classical and popular music, she also entertains the children with theme songs from their favorite TV programs. To all outward appearances, Frieda is a cheerful person, and few would suspect that she is depressed. "I am a gay depressive," she declares with the dramatic flair one would expect from a European concert pianist, "and I'm not referring to the sexual sense of the word."

What most people do not know is that for some time, Frieda has no longer enjoyed the many things that used to delight and enchant her. She has withdrawn from people and has not finished reading a book or been to a performance at the Kennedy Center for the past three years. Life feels very difficult. She is pressed for money, and everything seems like an effort. Her thoughts often turn to gloomy themes and she is beset by all sorts of imaginary fears. For example, on her recent visit to her doctor, she worried that she would get lost or trip in his garden. Even worse, she dwells at times on thoughts of taking an overdose of medications and being done with her suffering once and for all.

Frieda's history with antidepressants is an unhappy one. She compares herself to an overweight person who has tried a number of diets but has ended up heavier than she was at the beginning. She feels that every antidepressant she tried left her worse off than she was before. She claims to be the first person to give "a bad report on Prozac." She can't remember what the problems were with Zoloft and Wellbutrin, both of which she tried, with untoward effects. Effexor caused "brain activity while I was asleep—terrifying dreams" that disturbed her nights and left her exhausted during the day.

When St. John's wort began to garner attention in the media, Frieda read up on it in a Hungarian book of herbs and decided to try it. As she put it, "In Europe everybody knows about it. Americans always discover things hundreds of years later." Frieda discontinued the Effexor, and after ten days shifted to St. John's wort, 300 mg twice a day. This is the first antidepressant she has ever taken that has not bothered her with its side effects. She is highly circumspect about the reason for her improved sleep and energy level, wondering whether it might be due exclusively to being off Effexor as opposed to an effect of the herbal antidepressant. Her psychiatrist has recommended that she increase the dosage to see whether the improvement continues. In the meantime, her suicidal ideas have left her and she is guardedly optimistic that further positive developments may follow.

In the stories of the elderly people described here, we see many elements of how depression affects older people. As with Frieda, what we commonly think of as an essential element of depression, namely, depressed mood, may be missing in the elderly. Instead, there is a marked anhedonia, a loss of pleasure in things that were formerly interesting or were joyful activities. Physical symptoms such as difficulty with sleep, appetite or weight changes, and low energy levels are common symptoms of depression in older people and are important clues to the presence of a treatable condition. As we have seen, depression is often masked by many physical symptoms. In many of these depressed people, these physical difficulties cannot be adequately explained in terms of physical illnesses.

Many of the elderly people described here had reasons to be depressed, including bereavements, physical illnesses, and the loss of meaningful work. Nevertheless, it still paid to treat them medically despite these "explanations." Suicidal ideas are all too common in older depressed people and it is critical that these be viewed as symptoms of the illness and not dismissed as rational responses to life circumstances, no matter how reasonable they may appear to be to an outsider. Quite apart from the medical treatment of depression, whether with St. John's wort or another antidepressant, it is important that a depressed person be given the opportunity to discuss real life difficulties with an understanding and empathic person. Although there is no substitute for the loving support of friends and family, psychotherapy can be very helpful in this regard.

There are as yet no formal published studies on the use of St. John's wort in the elderly. Indeed, there are far fewer studies of any treatments of depression in the elderly than in younger and healthier populations. As the elderly become statistically and economically a more important demographic group, this situation is certain to be remedied. In the meantime, however, the very positive experiences of a growing number of physicians and patients with the use of St. John's wort to treat depression in the elderly—its apparent efficacy, ease of combination with other medications, and benign side-effect profile—are so encouraging that St. John's wort is surely worth considering for anyone who is elderly and depressed.

Part II

THE HERBAL WAY TO FEELING GOOD

A Practical Guide to the Use of St. John's Wort

8

DIAGNOSING YOUR OWN DEPRESSION

People often confuse clinical depression with sadness. That's a mistake. You can be sad without being clinically depressed and vice versa. Let's say, for example, that you have been rejected by a person you love, have been fired from your job, or have suffered a major setback in some project in which you have invested a lot of time and energy. It would be strange not to experience some feelings of sadness in the days or even weeks following such a reversal of fortune. But if such normal sadness is short-lived and not accompanied by some of the tell-tale signs of depression listed below, no doctor would diagnose you as being clinically depressed. You would expect to see the feelings of sadness diminish over days or weeks and be replaced by other feelings—relief, hopefulness, or even happiness, and, together with those feelings, optimistic thoughts. Maybe it wasn't such a great relationship and you're better off out of it. And the job wasn't necessarily that terrific, now that you think about it; some other job might suit you better. And as for the setback, it hurt, no question about it, but it wasn't critical—you take your licks, learn your lessons, and move on.

As you will see in the pages of this book, a capacity to get on with things is not a hallmark of depression. When you are depressed, you feel trapped and stuck. Solutions do not present themselves to you. It often seems as though there is no way out. Sadness by itself does not mean you are depressed, even though sadness is certainly one of the cardinal symptoms of depression. Often, this is not an ordinary sadness, focused on a single situation or event. Rather, it is a pervasive sadness that seems to settle on everything. The sadness can take over all other feelings, leaving little room for happiness, contentment, good humor, or even anger. But even though sadness is one of the most common symptoms of depression, it is also one of the easiest to connect with the condition. In our everyday language, a person might say "I feel sad" or "I feel depressed" interchangeably. In contrast, there are other symptoms that may be less obviously associated with depression but are nevertheless cardinal symptoms and signs of the condition. I call them the seven telltale signs of depression. It is easy to attribute these signs, correctly or incorrectly, to conditions other than depression. But when they are present, depression is one condition that should always be considered.

The Seven Telltale Signs of Depression

- running on empty
- nothing seems like fun anymore; life seems dreary
- putting yourself down
- failure—at work and in relationships
- biological disturbances—sleeping, eating, weight, and sex drive
- the future looks bleak
- life seems not worth living

Running on Empty

Not long ago newspapers reported that the president of Harvard University was unable to return to work. Amid speculation as to what might be wrong with him, his doctor issued a bulletin saying that he was exhausted from overwork. He was running on empty. Well, you don't have to be the president of Harvard University to know how that feels. I have encountered this symptom in depressed patients I have treated from all walks of life. I recall a highly skilled psychotherapist who was in such great demand because of his expertise that he received many more referrals than he could comfortably handle. Unfortunately, he was much more skillful at taking care of his patients than of himself and had a hard time disappointing his referral sources. He seriously overbooked his schedule, leaving much too little time for rest, exercise, and recreation. As a result, his depression was extremely difficult to treat. No matter what antidepressants I gave him, he always seemed to be running on empty.

Population studies in the United States suggest that depression is becoming more common with each successive generation, our youngest people being most frequently affected. No one knows why this is happening. One possible reason is the cost of upward mobility. As our society becomes increasingly sophisticated technologically, the newly created opportunities carry with them certain risks and hazards. Increasingly, there are businesses that stay open till all hours of the night. People take their computers on vacation with them so that they can plug into their E-mail and connect to the Internet from the most remote of places. They carry cellular phones and are always on call, wired in and connected to their business associates and customers. And businesses themselves, in an attempt to become more competitive, squeeze the most that they can out of each employee. One patient of mine, a pharmacist who supervised several pharmacies, kept being given more and more stores to supervise. Just as with the psychotherapist I mentioned, her depression was very hard to treat and only responded, finally and completely, when she quit her job.

The curious thing about depression, though, is that you can end up running on empty regardless of how great your burdens are in any objective sense. Each of us has our comfort zone in which we can function happily and efficiently, and each of us has our limit, beyond which our capacity to function breaks down. When someone becomes depressed, that breaking point has been exceeded. It does no good to debate whether or not you should be able to handle the level of stress. Regardless of the objective level of stress that you are currently under, if your capacity for handling that stress has been exceeded, you will feel as though you are running on empty and that may be an indication that you are clinically depressed, especially when it is combined with one or more of the other telltale signs of depression.

One of the hardest things to do when you are running on empty is to start new projects. New initiatives invariably require a new burst of energy, which is especially difficult to muster when you are down.

It is also important to remember that running on empty may be a symptom of other illnesses. Chronic infections, such as mononucleosis, may strip you of energy, as may many other medical disorders. Chronic fatigue syndrome (CFS) is a particularly vexing condition in which a low energy level is the cardinal and sometimes the only symptom. Low thyroid function and other hormonal conditions may also result in fatigue and low energy levels. Some of these conditions can be diagnosed by simple blood tests. This is one reason that, in the best of all possible worlds, you should get a medical evaluation before reaching a definitive diagnosis of depression. Or, if you don't choose to do that, reevaluate the situation if you try to treat your depression and it hasn't improved substantially within a month or two.

> If you have been running on empty for more than a few weeks, consider the possibility that you may be clinically depressed.

Nothing Seems Like Fun Anymore; Life Seems Dreary

Life is difficult. That is how M. Scott Peck begins *The Road Less Traveled*, one of the most successful books of all time. As he points out, that statement is one of the great, inescapable truths, which has been emphasized by philosophers since the time of the Buddha. Hard work, losses, injustices, illnesses, and poverty are among the problems that are part of our human condition. Despite these difficulties, however, the capacity of the human spirit to rise above them time and again has repeatedly been observed. Victor Frankl survived one of the greatest horrors of our modern era or, perhaps, of all time—the Holocaust—and went on to write his classic inspirational work, *Man's Search for Meaning*, in which he emphasized our capacity to find significance and value even in the most horrible of circumstances. He regarded such an ability to preserve a sense of purpose and meaning as essential to survival.

Depressed people lose their capacity to see meaning and significance in their lives. A religious person when depressed may feel cut off from God, a particularly distressing loss at a time when spiritual comfort may be most deeply needed. In such a spiritual void, the depressed person may naturally feel that there is very little purpose in living.

Related to our ability to find a sense of meaning and purpose in life is our capacity to enjoy ourselves and have fun. We can see this ability at play even in the midst of all sorts of difficulties. Poor people retain their ability to celebrate, as anyone can see who has walked through the impoverished neighborhoods of some European town during a festival for a saint or at carnival time. Even very hardworking people take time out for recreation. When difficult times let up, even for a short interval, the ability to have fun pops up again like the crocuses that sprout their shoots and flowers after a long winter.

All of these normal abilities are the opposite of what we see in depression. Even in the midst of plenty—enough money, good physical health, supportive friends and family—the depressed person is unable to have a good time. This inability to enjoy life can come on insidiously and it may take awhile to realize that you are not enjoying life as you used to. Sometimes this recognition is triggered by returning to a place you've been before or an activity you used to relish and realizing that you don't have the same feelings or enthusiasm for it that you once had. Sometimes friends will ask you what the matter is. You just don't seem to be enjoying yourself as you used to. Suddenly, or gradually, you realize that nothing feels like fun anymore. As one of my patients put it, depression is like an unwelcome guest who follows you around your house and just won't go away. The formal clinical term for this state is "anhedonia," which means the inability to experience pleasure.

Life feels dreary. Sometimes this dreariness is experienced through the senses. Colors seem less bright than they did before. The world may look gray or dark where formerly it was full of vivid colors. Whatever it is that you may have loved—music, dancing, movies—now feels like a drag. In this way, depression is like a thief that robs you of the joy of living. This is another reason not to delay in treating it so that you can reclaim the ability to experience joy once again.

> If nothing seems like fun anymore and life seems dreary, and this has been going on for more than a few weeks, consider the possibility that you may be clinically depressed.

Putting Yourself Down

Self-criticism is part of the way we regulate the quality of our performance in the various aspects of our lives—our work, our relationships, and even our pastimes. We are constantly judging ourselves. This often begins first thing in the morning when we look in the mirror. "How do I look today? Are there bags under my eyes? Is my hair okay? Do these clothes fit properly? Do they suit me?" Or when we step onto the bathroom scale. "Have I gained a pound or two? Did I overeat last night? Or drink too much?" Either the question is answered or the answer is deferred. And so it goes on, for many of us, throughout the day.

At the office you might ask: "How did I handle that last meeting? Did I say the right thing in the right way? How did it go over with the boss, the client, the organization? Was the product up to my usual standard?" A parent may ask, "Is my child doing okay and, if not, am I to blame?" A homemaker may ask, "Am I keeping up with the housework or taking care of the home properly?" In our relationships we may ask, "Am I a good enough wife, husband, or lover?" or "Am I getting the love or attention I want and need?" And so it goes. We ask, we judge, we reach conclusions. This is an important ongoing process because it is a feedback loop by which we calibrate the quality of our lives and the basis for making changes or corrections so that our needs are met and we feel good about ourselves and the way things are going.

In depression, though, this whole process is disturbed. We see ourselves through a distorting lens. In the extreme case, the depressed person feels ugly and a failure in all the areas that matter. Such judgments are made more confusing by the fact that the disorder itself causes us to fail in many ways, as I describe below. Even so, it is typical of a depressed person to exaggerate these failures far beyond what is reasonable and accurate. And it is this tendency toward extreme exaggeration that is a major telltale sign of depression. The conclusions reached by a depressed person, far from being an accurate take on reality, are in fact yet another manifestation of this multifaceted disorder. "I am a terrible housewife; nothing I ever do turns out right," or "I'm a terrible mother; my children would be better off without me," or "I'm no good at all at what I do; I deserve to be fired" are common laments. The distortions may be projected into the future, as in "I'll never amount to anything" and "I have fooled people into believing I'm competent and sooner or later I'll be discovered to be an imposter." Sometimes the distortions are so gross that they would almost seem comical were it not for the pain and distress of the person experiencing them. For example, one colleague quotes a patient of his as saying, "I am the most unimportant person in the world."

Whenever you find yourself using exaggerated phraseology in connection with yourself, such as "the most," "the worst," or "the least," you should suspect yourself of being the victim of distorted perceptions and very possibly suffering from depression. Such distortions have been a focus of one of the most successful forms of psychotherapy for depression, namely, cognitive therapy, in which a person's distortions are systematically challenged and subjected to scrutiny by using the patient's capacity to reason, which is often intact in people suffering from depression. Cognitive therapists have actually shown that such rigorous challenging of aberrant perceptions and ideas can correct not only the distorted thinking of the depressed person but can also result in a beneficial effect on the person's mood.

> If you are in the habit of putting yourself down or constantly seeing yourself in the worst possible light, and this has been going on for more than a few weeks, consider the possibility that you may be clinically depressed.

Failure—At Work and in Relationships

Depression cuts into a person's ability to function so that some of the failure that he or she perceives does have a basis in reality. Mental processes slow down and it is difficult to concentrate, to focus, or to get things done. Work inevitably suffers, chores remain undone, things get botched up, leaving you with feelings of failure and inadequacy, much of which may be exaggerated but some of which may be true. It is easy to forget how competent you have been at other times and how much you have accomplished before. All these things seem insignificant when you are depressed. Dr. Kay Redfield Jamison, in her wonderful memoir, *An Unquiet Mind*, describes the difficulties in thinking she experienced during one of her depressions:

> Everything—every thought, word, movement—was an effort. Everything that once was sparkling now was flat. I seemed to myself to be dull, boring, inadequate, thick brained, unlit, unresponsive, chill skinned, bloodless, and sparrow drab. I doubted, completely, my ability to do anything well. It seemed as though my mind had slowed down and burned out to the point of being virtually useless. The wretched, convoluted, and pathetically

confused mass of gray worked only well enough to tor-
ment me with a litany of my inadequacies and short-
comings in character, and to taunt me with the total, the
desperate, hopelessness of it all.

This description of severe depression conveys many aspects
of a depressed person's thinking. In the years that followed the
depression described above, Dr. Jamison went on to succeed
enormously as a psychologist, researcher, and writer, but such
a future is unthinkable when you are in the depths of a depression. It is important to realize how misleading the conclusions
reached in a state of depression can be.

When you are depressed, all the skills that are involved in
working productively may be impaired. Work involves motivation, from the moment you get up in the morning, travel to
work, and set about tackling your job, right until the workday
is over. Motivation is critical at every step along the way.
Depression can present an obstacle at each of these steps, turning a job that previously might have been easy into a mountain-
ous ordeal. All work involves thinking—concentrating, remembering, and making connections between ideas—and all of
these suffer when one is depressed. Everything takes longer
and is more laborious. Small wonder that one feels exhausted
by the end of the workday. Social interactions are difficult. It is
hard to initiate contact with others and telephone messages
remain unanswered. This compounds a depressed person's
sense of isolation and failure. Finally, all the small pleasures
that help move along one's work—joking with colleagues, the
enjoyment of one's own competency, and the satisfaction of a
job well done—are absent from the work life of a depressed
person.

Failure is also experienced in one's personal life.
Relationships require a capacity to attend to another person
and an ability to feel engaged with that person, both of which
are sorely deficient in depression. Others may well feel put off
and withdraw in response to the reclusiveness of a depressed
person.

If you find you have been failing at work or in your personal relationships in a way that has not always been typical for you, and this has been going on for more than a few weeks, consider the possibility that you may be clinically depressed.

Biological Disturbances—Sleeping, Eating, Weight, and Sex Drive

One major difference between sadness and depression is that the latter is often accompanied by changes in biological functioning. These biological changes are among the most reliable telltale signs of depression, and when doctors and therapists look for depression, they carefully inquire into changes in sleeping, eating, weight, and sex drive. You should certainly pay special attention to these important behavioral functions in evaluating whether you are depressed and, if so, how severely depressed you are.

In depression, sleep is often disrupted. Some depressed people have trouble falling asleep; others toss and turn or wake during the night; and early morning waking, often with difficulty returning to sleep, is very common. Sleep doesn't seem to have its usual renewing properties and people are often left feeling tired during the day and desperate at night for sleep that stubbornly refuses to arrive. Some depressed patients sleep too much, at times for hours each day more than is normal for them, and yet, once again, find that no matter how much they sleep, they still don't end up feeling refreshed.

These two patterns of sleep disruption—insomnia and oversleeping—may signal two distinct types of depression, one representing a state of hypervigilant overarousal and the other a state of torpid underarousal. These patterns may reflect exaggerations of different types of responses to stress.

When people (or animals, for that matter) are stressed, a part of the brain known as the hypothalamus activates a stress-response system, which results in the release of certain hormones from the adrenal glands, particularly cortisol. In addition, the fight-and-flight part of the nervous system, known as the sympathetic nervous system, is activated. These changes result in arousal and vigilance, qualities that are necessary for combating stress, and are associated with decreases in sleep and appetite. The type of depression associated with decreased sleep and appetite and weight loss may represent an exaggeration of these arousal responses. Evidence to support this theory is found in the form of elevated cortisol levels in the circulation and other signs of overactivity of the stress-responsive hormonal system in these depressed patients.

The heightened arousal and vigilance that are part of our normal response to stress should be limited in time in order to be most effective. Ideally, such responses should kick in following a stressful situation, such as the loss of a loved one, a physical challenge, or an important deadline, and should subside when the stress has been successfully handled or resolved. In depression, the stress response may be triggered by either a definable stress or by some unknown factor, but whatever its original trigger, it then takes on a life of its own, persisting long after the stress is over. Consider, for example, a person susceptible to depression who is told that he has lost a large sum of money on the stock market, whereupon he plummets into a deep depression. If that same person is told a week later that his stockbroker has made a mistake and that he has actually made a lot of money instead of losing it, will his depression immediately disappear? Probably not. Such is the nature of depression that once it gets going, it can continue indefinitely. As you can imagine, this wears the system down and the person is left feeling exhausted and depleted.

The second type of depression—the one associated with oversleeping, overeating, and weight gain—may represent an exaggeration of the energy-conserving responses seen frequently in animals. The hibernating bear, for example, goes into a state of low activity and torpor designed to conserve its energy and resources. Such slowing down of bodily activities enables the bear to make it through a winter of severe weather and scarce food. Most people with seasonal affective disorder (SAD), many of whom compare themselves to hibernating bears, experience this second type of depression and tend to oversleep, as well as overeat and gain weight, during their winter depressions.

Withdrawal and seclusion, as part of the recovery process, often occur in animals as a response to stress or injury. An injured lion, for example, may retreat to its lair until its wounds have healed before venturing back out into the savannas and exposing itself to the dangers of the wild. An infant monkey separated from its mother initially goes into a state where it cries out pitifully, which was termed the stage of protest by John Bowlby, a pioneer in the area of separation and loss. Later, the infant goes into another state that Bowlby called detachment, where it withdraws from contact with other animals. It has been suggested that these stages are ways in which the animal adapts to the loss of its mother. Initially, it makes noises, which would have the function of attracting the attention of the mother, who might not be far away. After a while, however, if the mother has not responded, she might well have been killed and the infant's cries would be more likely to elicit the attention of a predator. In the course of evolution, it has probably proven far more adaptive for the infant to go into a state of withdrawal at this point and wait until another parental figure might chance to come along. There is a final stage that has been described in such separated infant monkeys—a stage of reattachment, whereby the infant will reattach to a new parental figure that might arrive. Over the millennia, certain adaptive behavioral changes to injury and loss have evolved so as to maximize the chance of survival. It has been suggested that some of the behavioral and physical symptoms of depression may represent disturbances of the normal biological systems responsible for mediating such adaptive responses.

When an animal is stressed, the emphasis is on survival, as well it should be. Having sex is the last thing that will be on that animal's mind. And so it is that with the depressed person, the sex drive diminishes and may shut off completely. Every aspect of sexual functioning may be affected—arousal, enjoyment of sex, and the capacity to function. Needless to say, this does not much help the self-esteem of the depressed person, which is already at a very low ebb.

So we see that in depression there may be an exaggeration of some of our very useful responses to the stresses and challenges that life deals us. When these responses—such as hyper-vigilance or excessive withdrawal—go too far, they hinder rather than help our ability to adapt. They continue for much too long and we are unable to turn them off by an act of will.

If your sleeping, eating, weight control, and interest in sex are disturbed, and this has been going on for more than a few weeks, consider the possibility that you may be suffering from depression.

The Future Looks Bleak

Just as depression tends to cast a gray pall over everything in your world and in yourself, so there is an irresistible tendency to project that gloomy view into the future. The depressed person will always find something to be pessimistic about. And as with one's view of the present, these gloomy predictions are often without any reasonable basis in reality. And even when there are problems in a person's life, there are many different ways to look at the future. A person with cancer, for example, may have a very optimistic and upbeat view of the future, whereas a depressed person in perfectly good physical condition may be full of gloomy predictions about his health. In fact, in one research study, patients who had suffered from both cancer and depression were asked to rate which of their two conditions involved greater suffering. They rated depression as the more painful of the two conditions. In summary, there is not generally a very close correlation between the realistic prospects for a person's future and how a depressed person is likely to view it. Pessimism is a cardinal symptom of depression.

If the future seems bleak and gloomy to you, and this has been going on for more than a few weeks, consider the possibility that you may be depressed.

Life Seems Not Worth Living

As you can imagine, with all the symptoms I have just listed, including a grim and bleak view of your present situation and future prospects, a depressed person may easily reach the conclusion—or at least entertain the possibility—that life is not worth living. This symptom of depression, known to the clinician as "suicidal ideation," is a very troublesome one. If you are experiencing any such ideas, please do yourself and everyone who cares about you a great favor and consult a physician without delay. Depression is a condition in which hope is in short supply, and one way to get an infusion of hope is to reach out to those who may be able to guide you out of your dark place. Your physician is a logical first port of call in such an attempt to reach out. But if, for any reason, it is difficult for you to talk to your physician about the problem, tell *someone*— a family member, a friend, or even someone on a crisis hot line. Suicidal ideation is not a symptom that anyone ought to have to suffer alone.

As depression deepens, suicidal ideation may progress to passive suicidal longings, which may be accompanied by lack of self-care or carelessness. A depressed woman may feel a lump in her breast while taking a shower and may say to herself, "So what if it's cancer? It would probably be all for the best anyway." Another depressed person might cross the road carelessly and, in the back of his mind, be thinking, "Well, if I get run over, what loss will that be to anyone?"

Matters become even more serious when suicidal ideas begin to gel into actual plans and, even more so, when actions are taken to put these plans into effect. It might seem unnecessary to say that if someone you know or love should mention suicidal ideas or plans to you, these should always be taken seriously. Unfortunately, it is still all too common for people to minimize the seriousness of such communications. The idea that if someone tells you he is considering suicide he is unlikely to act on it is a very dangerous myth. Such divulgences should always be heard as a communication of despair, which may or may not involve immediate danger but which always warrant serious attention. At the very least it is an expression of severe mental anguish.

> If you think that life is not worth living or have any thoughts or plans to end your life, you are very, very likely to be depressed. Please don't delay in getting professional help for this problem.

The Clinical Diagnosis of Depression

The diagnosis of depression has always been—and continues to be—made largely on the basis of a person's subjective history. Although a skillful clinician will see traces of depression in a person's face, observe sluggishness or agitation in the body's movements, and hear the slow cadence of the voice, it is the depressed person's own story that will carry the day in making the diagnosis. A few decades ago there was great optimism that a laboratory test for depression could readily be found. No such luck. For better or for worse, in your recollections of how you have been feeling and your accurate take on your present mood, you hold the key to determining whether or not you are depressed. What the skilled clinician does is to organize these recollections and evaluate whether or not they meet modern diagnostic criteria for depression.

I remember well, before modern systems of diagnosis had been developed, how the question of diagnosis would be debated in teaching hospitals. A patient would be interviewed and there would be discussion to and fro as to the exact diagnosis. Finally the professor would opine as to whether he (and yes, it was almost always a man) thought that the patient was depressed or not. And his opinion would prevail because he was the boss. Well, clearly, that was a most unsatisfactory state of affairs. For clinical, research, and, more recently, insurance purposes, it became necessary to define depression.

The latest diagnostic classification system put out by the American Psychiatric Association is called the *DSM-IV,* a handbook referred to by insurance companies and others to determine a person's clinical diagnosis. Each diagnosis is given a specific code number, which may be familiar to you from your medical bill. The diagnosis for many psychiatric conditions, including clinical depression, referred to officially as major depressive disorder, was reached by the so-called Chinese menu approach. In Chinese restaurants, the fixed-price menus permit you to have a certain number of items from column A, a certain number from column B, and so on. That's how it is with the *DSM-IV* criteria for major depressive disorder, which I have modified and listed below. It is worth checking out whether you meet the criteria for major depressive disorder. It is important to remember that these are strict criteria. If you do not meet these criteria, that does not mean that you are not depressed and might not still benefit from St. John's wort and the other remedies mentioned in this book.

DSM-IV Criteria for Major Depressive Disorder

A. Five (or more) of the following symptoms have been present for two solid weeks. This is different from your usual functioning. At least one of the symptoms must be either (1) depressed mood or (2) loss of interest or pleasure.

1. depressed mood most of the day, nearly every day, either experienced by yourself or observed by others

2. markedly diminished interest or pleasure in all, or almost all, activities, most of the day, nearly every day

3. significant weight loss when not dieting, or weight gain, or decrease or increase in appetite nearly every day

4. sleeping too much or too little nearly every day

5. being agitated or depressed to such a degree that others could notice it—not just internal feelings of restlessness or being slowed down

6. fatigue or loss of energy nearly every day

7. feelings of worthlessness or excessive or inappropriate guilt nearly every day—more than just feeling guilty because your depression doesn't enable you to function adequately

8. decreased ability to think or concentrate, or difficulty making decisions, nearly every day

9. recurrent thoughts of death (not just fear of dying), recurrent ideas of suicide or attempting or planning suicide

AND

B. These symptoms cause significant distress or impairment in your social, occupational, or other important areas of functioning.

AND

C. The symptoms are not directly due to the physical effects of medications, drugs, or alcohol, nor are the result of a medical condition, such as underactive thyroid functioning.

Now, many people who feel quite depressed do not exactly fit into the *DSM-IV* criteria for major depression. The diagnostic schema allows for those types of depression as well. These include briefer depressions that occur premenstrually (premenstrual dysphoric disorder), milder depressions (minor depressive disorder), and recurrent depressions that can be very severe even though they may last for only a few days at a time (recurrent brief depressive disorder). The good news is that all of these depressions, as well as those that accompany medical conditions or may be associated with drugs and alcohol, may be helped by the same treatments that are helpful for major depression.

One diagnosis, which has its own code in *DSM-IV*, is "dysthymic disorder," a milder form of depression that causes a great deal of misery because of its chronic nature. I have modified the *DSM-IV* criteria for dysthymic disorder and have listed them below.

DSM-IV Criteria for Dysthymic Disorder

A. Depressed mood for most of the day, for more days than not, either experienced by yourself or observed by others, for at least two years.

AND

B. Presence, while depressed, of two or more of the following:

1. poor appetite or overeating

2. insomnia or sleeping too much

3. fatigue or low energy

4. low self-esteem

5. poor concentration or difficulty making decisions

6. feelings of hopelessness

AND

C. During a two-year period, you have never been without the symptoms in A or B for more than two months at a time.

AND

D. The symptoms are not due to the direct physical effects of medications, drugs, or alcohol or to a general medical condition, such as underactive thyroid functioning.

As you read through the criteria, it will become obvious that they are somewhat arbitrary. What if you were free of symptoms for two and a half months? Does that mean that you are not dysthymic or wouldn't benefit from treatment? Although systematic diagnostic schemas have been useful for standardizing diagnoses for research and other purposes, the seasoned clinician and the savvy patient should realize that diagnosis is not a precise science and not get too hung up on whether someone exactly meets the criteria or not before deciding on whether and how to treat. It is clear that when we are dealing with depression, in all its forms, we are dealing with a continuum, with happy, normal mood at the one end and serious depression at the other and all sorts of gradations in between. The same treatments that help the more severe forms of depression will generally also help the milder forms and vice versa. The most important determinants of whether or not you seek and receive treatment are therefore how bad you feel and whether you are willing to reach out for help.

How Bad Is Your Depression?

One point that bears repeating is that depression exists on a spectrum of severity, ranging from mild feelings of low energy, sadness, and being stressed out to full-blown suicidal melancholia. It is obviously very important to determine the severity of the depression in order to treat it properly. This determination has relevance not only for the use of St. John's wort but as an overall guide to optimal treatment. As I have mentioned, the strongest evidence for the benefits of St. John's wort come from studies of mild to moderate depression. If depression is mild, or even moderate, it may be reasonable to try a home remedy before seeking medical help, at least for a limited period of time. Severe depression, on the other hand, should be regarded as a medical emergency and should be treated by a physician without delay. In such cases, it would pay to start out with one of the more conventional antidepressants, which have a more proven track record in the treatment of severe depression.

One way to distinguish between mild to moderate depression and severe depression is to examine how well you are doing in those areas of life that are important to you. How are things going in your relationships, at the job, and in your ability to enjoy your leisure time? If they are going badly, this might be a clue that your depression is more serious than you realize. When considering the impact of depression on a person's life, it is extremely difficult to disentangle cause and effect. A depressed person is quite likely to perceive the mood problem as being a result of all that is not going well in his or her life when, actually, the reverse may be true. Are you depressed because of a bad marriage, a bad job, and difficult life circumstances, or are these difficulties occurring because you are depressed? Given the impossibility of answering this question with any degree of certainty, it is best to assume that the depression is the culprit that is souring the rest of your life because it's usually the easiest thing to fix. So in judging the degree of your depression, consider how things are going in the various compartments of your life.

Reading through the list of symptoms in the major depression criteria listed on pages 104–105 will also provide you with a guide to the severity of your depression. In general, the more symptoms you have, the more severely depressed you are. Each symptom can in itself be measured according to its severity. In fact, that is how researchers measure depression—by asking about the severity of a large number of depressive symptoms, giving each symptom a score, and then adding up the symptom scores to obtain a total. It is worth asking yourself how bad your various depressive symptoms are, and if you find that they are cutting into your functioning to any significant degree, then you should certainly consult a doctor. The following summary should help you to determine how seriously affected you are along the depressive spectrum. In a later chapter I discuss when and how best to choose a suitable doctor.

A Guide to Evaluating Where You Fit on the Depressive Spectrum

Level of Depression	Symptoms	Effects
stressed out; down in the dumps; under the weather	fatigue; mild anxiety; lack of zest; less fun than usual	others may well not notice anything amiss; no effect on functioning
mild depression	a few symptoms listed above, but none are severe	slightly diminished quality of life, productivity, or creativity; you notice this but others would probably not
moderate depression	meet the criteria for *DSM-IV* major depression listed above	significant impact on functioning in work or relationships; significant impact on physical functioning; it is, however, possible in many cases to function well in certain respects, making others unaware of how bad you are feeling; those close to you are likely to be aware that something is amiss

A Guide to Evaluating Where You Fit on the Depressive Spectrum *(continued)*

Level of Depression	Symptoms	Effects
severe depression	meet the criteria for *DSM-IV* major depression listed above; any suicidal ideas or intentions	it is difficult to function adequately at work or in relationships; significant impact on physical functioning; can be a threat to your relationship, your job, or, if you are suicidal, to life itself; others are very likely to be aware that something is amiss and to be concerned about you

Both moderate and severe levels of depression would be considered to be clinical, or major, depression. If you fit into either of those categories, you should certainly seek out the help of a competent professional. This does not mean that St. John's wort should not be part of the treatment plan, if not initially, then somewhere down the line.

If you are suffering from the two less severe levels on the depressive spectrum, it may be appropriate to treat yourself at least initially with St. John's wort and to consult a professional only if your attempts to help yourself are unsuccessful.

What Is the Shape of the Monkey on Your Back?

Depression has often been compared to a beast. It *is* a beastly condition. Sir Winston Churchill called it his black dog, conveying how it seems to attack from outside and overwhelm us with gloom. In everyday terms, we speak of having a monkey on the back. But depression is a monkey that comes in different shapes. And it is worth considering these different shapes because it helps us understand and treat the type of depression in question.

Depression can come as a single episode or be recurrent. When recurrent episodes consist only of depressions, the condition is termed unipolar. Bipolar disorder, on the other hand, means that depressed episodes are interspersed with manic or hypomanic (a bit less severe than manic) episodes, when a person becomes excessively activated, overtalkative, and sped up. Manias and hypomanias can cause major problems in their own right, a full discussion of which goes beyond the scope of this book. An important thing to bear in mind, however, if one has a tendency to bipolar disorder, is that all antidepressant treatments have been shown to be capable of inducing manic or hypomanic episodes. So far, to my knowledge, there have been no published reports of St. John's wort inducing a manic or hypomanic episode, but as it is an active antidepressant treatment, it would come as no surprise if it were capable of causing such episodes in susceptible individuals.

Recovery from depression may be complete. Alternatively, depressions may be superimposed on a dysthymic disorder, in which case recovery is not complete but the remission of the more serious depression may return the unfortunate individual to the chronic state of misery that is the hallmark of dysthymia. This type of depression has also been referred to as double depression, indicating that a really bad depression can be superimposed on a milder, more chronic, underlying depression.

Depressions may take on a seasonal pattern. The most common type of seasonal pattern is marked by winter depressions, which improve in the summertime, a condition known as seasonal affective disorder (SAD). Some people with SAD do not recover completely in the summertime although their depressions may become much less severe. In other words, they have a type of double depression. Such a seasonal pattern is worth noting, since it suggests that the winter depressions may respond favorably to light therapy. Some people have regularly recurring seasonal depressions at times of year other than the winter, particularly in the summer.

People with recurrent brief depression (RBD) have frequent depressive episodes that usually last between two and four days. Despite their brevity, these depressions cause a great deal of pain and studies show that about a quarter of these individuals have attempted suicide at some time in their past. I once asked a patient with this type of depression how depressed he had been, on average. He replied that on average he had not been very depressed at all, but pointed out that I had asked the question in the wrong way, noting, "You can drown in a river that is only six inches deep on average if it has some very deep places in it." And that is how it feels to have recurrent brief depressions. All of a sudden you can feel as though you are drowning. It is only recently that much attention has been focused on RBD even though it appears to be quite common. So far, no systematic studies have shown much benefit from antidepressant medications for this disorder and no studies of St. John's wort have as yet been undertaken for this condition.

At this point, you should be able to identify whether you have the symptoms of depression, how severe these symptoms are, and whether they fall into some definable pattern. The next question is what to do about it. Should you consider going to a doctor? Is St. John's wort worth a try and, if so, how should you go about using it? These are some of the questions I tackle in the following chapters.

9

DEVELOPING A GAME PLAN FOR USING ST. JOHN'S WORT TO TREAT DEPRESSION

My goal in this chapter is to provide a key to the chapters that follow as well as an overview of how to set about using St. John's wort. This chapter is intended as a guide to developing a game plan for the treatment of depressive symptoms with the herbal remedy.

Those considering the use of St. John's wort fall into one of two categories. Either they are not currently being treated with antidepressants, or they are. I deal with each of these situations separately, as shown below.

If You Are Considering Starting St. John's Wort for the First Time, It Is Worth Asking Yourself These Questions

> Am I mildly blue, stressed out, and down in the dumps or actually clinically depressed? (See chapter 8 to help you decide.)

> Should I consider consulting a doctor? (See chapter 10 to help you decide.)

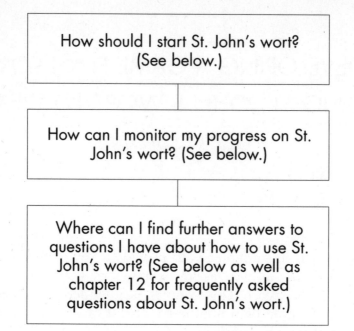

How should I start St. John's wort?
(See below.)

How can I monitor my progress on St.
John's wort? (See below.)

Where can I find further answers to
questions I have about how to use St.
John's wort? (See below as well as
chapter 12 for frequently asked
questions about St. John's wort.)

If You Are Not Currently Being Treated for Depression and Are Considering Starting St. John's Wort for the First Time, Consider Which of the Following Describes You Best

Are you:

stressed or feeling mildly blue, down in the dumps, or under the weather

suffering from clinical depression, also known as major depressive disorder, or dysthymia

somewhere in between (1) and (2) above

severely depressed

(See pages 103–110 to help you decide.)

Depression is not an all-or-none phenomenon like pregnancy, but exists in a whole range of different degrees and across a spectrum that goes from feeling slightly blue to being suicidally melancholic. Clearly, the degree of urgency and the appropriate steps to take in addressing the condition vary greatly depending on its severity. I will try to give you some further pointers to help you choose which category best fits you or someone you care about, but clearly it is a judgment call and it is wise to err on the side of caution.

1. Suggestions for those who are

- mildly blue

- stressed out

- under the weather

- down in the dumps

An old advertisement for an over-the-counter cold medication observed that you can't take every cold to a doctor and proceeded to recommend the medicine in question. The ad was right. It is not economically or logistically sensible to go to the doctor with every cold—or, for that matter, whenever you feel blue, down in the dumps, or lacking in energy and pep. On the other hand, a case of pneumonia should always be taken to a doctor—and promptly—and that applies to serious depression as well. And just as we have guidelines to help us distinguish between a cold and pneumonia, so we can distinguish between serious depression and feeling mildly out of sorts. In the mildly blue, stressed-out, under-the-weather category, I would put those whose symptoms are not seriously interfering with their work, personal relationships, or other aspects of their functioning. Also, the problem should not have been going on for too long, not more, say, than for a couple of months.

If you think you qualify for this very mild category, I suggest that you read about the symptoms and level of depression anyway because depressed people are often not very good at recognizing how depressed they are, and they are not alone in this regard. Statistics indicate that in a very great proportion of cases even doctors fail to recognize and treat depression properly. If professionals underestimate depression to this extent, laypeople can surely be forgiven for doing the same. Because many of the symptoms of depression do not actually involve sadness or depressed mood, but, rather, are physical symptoms, they are easily attributed to other conditions. In addition, depressed people often believe that their problems are due exclusively to influences from the outside world rather than some internal problem. This set of beliefs may be associated with a fear of acknowledging that "there may be something wrong with me," and a pessimism about being able to correct the problem. In fact, the opposite is often true, as it may be easier to correct problems that stem from within yourself than those that arise in the outside world, over which you may have very little control. So if you look through the list of symptoms and criteria for clinical depression and find that you are more markedly affected than you thought you were, this is no cause for despair, nor any reason to believe that you might not benefit from St. John's wort. It does mean that it is worth consulting a doctor, however, for all the reasons listed elsewhere in this book (see chapter 10).

If, after reflection, you feel that you are not clinically depressed, but simply overstressed or mildly down in the dumps, you may also benefit from a trial of St. John's wort. It is always important, of course, to address any underlying causes of your unhappiness in addition to taking the herbal remedy. Be sure to check out the suggestions listed in the chapter on adopting an antidepressant lifestyle to round out your treatment program.

Starting St. John's Wort: Getting the Dose Right

Since the target dosage in most of the antidepressant studies of mild to moderate depression has been 900 mg of hypericum per day, that is a reasonable dose to aim for. Tablets or capsules of St. John's wort or hypericum generally come in 150- or 300-mg dosages. The Kira brand of St. John's wort which, for reasons that I discuss later, is the one I recommend most highly, comes in only the 300-mg dosage, at least in the United States. Whenever I start someone on an antidepressant, I always begin with a low dose and increase the dosage somewhat gradually until the final, or target, dose is reached. The reason for this is that some people are very sensitive to medications and it is often not possible to predict who will be very sensitive and who will not. An average dose of an antidepressant may be far too much for such a person to tolerate, especially when just beginning the medication. If a highly sensitive person starts right out with an "average" dose of an antidepressant without building up to the final target dosage, unpleasant side effects may result and the person may be disinclined to ever try the medication again. So I would rather err on the side of moving a little too slowly. In practice, this means that I start a person on 300 mg of hypericum once a day for two or three days, then twice a day for two or three days, then three times a day. In older people, say, over sixty, I would proceed even more gradually.

If unpleasant side effects should develop, I slow down this progression, always working within the patient's comfort zone. In other words, if you are uncomfortable with one or two tablets of hypericum per day, don't move up the dosage until the side effects dissipate, as they generally will. Be sure to listen to what your body is telling you. Discomfort of any sort is a signal for you to slow down. In some sensitive people, including the elderly, a final dose of less than 900 mg a day, such as 600 mg, may work best.

- Be sure to take the hypericum with meals, as this minimizes the chances of developing indigestion or abdominal discomfort, which may occur in certain people on the herbal remedy.

- I recommend taking St. John's wort twice or three times a day rather than as a single dosage. That is how it has been administered in most research studies and it minimizes the likelihood of side effects.

Monitoring Your Progress on St. John's Wort

How can you monitor your progress on St. John's wort? The answer to this might seem obvious. Surely the medication either works or it doesn't. What is there to monitor? you might ask. Well, it is not always so clear-cut when a problem is relatively subtle to start with or when the response is modest or partial. I always find it useful to keep an eye on what are known as the target symptoms—those presenting problems that are part of the reason why someone is seeking help in the first place. We measure whether an antidepressant is working or not by focusing on changes in the target symptoms. In the case of someone with mild symptoms of depression or stress, such target symptoms might be a lack of the usual enjoyment or enthusiasm for life, decreased energy, anxiety, or sleep difficulties. It is worth listing those target symptoms that are most bothersome to you and observing each week whether you can detect any change in them. A log such as the one provided below can be helpful in tracking your progress as measured by the scale provided on the following page.

Log for Monitoring Effects of St. John's Wort on Target Symptoms of Depression

Target Symptom (e.g., anxiety, low energy, etc.)	Baseline and Weeks 1 through 6						
	Baseline	Week 1	Week 2	Week 3	Week 4	Week 5	Week 6

Scale:

0 = no change   −1 = a little worse

1 = a little better   −2 = quite a bit worse

2 = quite a bit better −3 = a lot worse

3 = a lot better

4 = completely better

I have been impressed with the highly variable time course of response to St. John's wort. Some people report feeling better within days of beginning the herbal remedy whereas for others the response is far slower and more subtle. A proper trial takes at least five to six weeks. If you are still feeling down in the dumps or overstressed at that point, I suggest that you take some further step, such as consulting with a physician or a therapist. If you are feeling better and are not suffering any significant side effects, you may wish to stay on the St. John's wort regimen for a further three months before thinking of tapering it and determining whether you can maintain the gains without any further help from the herbal remedy. If you experience unacceptable side effects, feel free to lower the dosage and see whether you still feel better. You can always raise it again later if you need to.

2. Suggestions for Those Suffering from Clinical Depression, Also Known As Major Depressive Disorder, or Dysthymia

Major depressive disorder and dysthymia are officially recognized conditions, which are defined on pages 104–107. Major depressive disorder disrupts one's capacity to function and enjoy one's life. Although even minor levels of depression can interfere with productivity, creativity, and the quality of one's relationships, in major depressions these functions are disrupted to an even greater degree. A major depression is, by definition, reasonably severe and lasts for at least two weeks. Dysthymia is less severe in terms of the number of symptoms required for its diagnosis but is, by definition, rather chronic and, as such, also exacts a toll on one's life. The criteria listed on pages 104–106 can help you decide whether you might be suffering from one of these two conditions. If you are, I do recommend that you consult a doctor, but this certainly does not mean that you cannot take—or benefit from—St. John's wort. Involving a doctor in your care can be challenging, especially when you are dealing with an "alternative" treatment such as the use of an herbal product. To guide you as to how best to involve an appropriate doctor in helping you with your problem (or in extricating yourself from an inappropriate one), consult chapter 10.

The directions for getting started on St. John's wort are the same as those described above. If you experience no response within five weeks, however, and are experiencing no unacceptable side effects, you may consider pushing up the dosage to four, five, or even six 300-mg tablets per day. Maintain the three-times-a-day dosing schedule, remembering to take St. John's wort with food, and wait at least three or four days between dosage increments. There is a range of effective dosages for all other antidepressants and there is no reason to believe that such a range would not apply to St. John's wort as well. Sometimes a full clinical response to an antidepressant will not be observed until the dosage is pushed into the higher levels of the accepted therapeutic range. So far there has been only one published clinical trial in which six 300-mg tablets were given per day (a total daily dosage of 1,800 mg). According to the researcher in charge of the study, levels of side effects were not noticeably higher for the 1,800-mg-per-day dosage than he has generally observed when treating people with the more conventional 900-mg-per-day dosage.

Unless the depression is severe, it is quite reasonable to use St. John's wort as a first-line treatment, in combination with other methods of promoting an antidepressant lifestyle, as outlined in chapter 11. Monitor your symptoms as described above. In addition, those suffering from major depression may find the more extensive log on pages 217–218 a helpful guide in monitoring your level of depression. Since it is a daily log, as opposed to the weekly log provided on page 118, it enables you to get a more fine-grained sense of your mood control and helps you recognize influences that may have an adverse or beneficial effect on your mood. Subtle mood cycles can also become apparent and their pattern may suggest certain specific types of treatment.

Once again, allow five to six weeks for the treatment to work. If it doesn't work by that time, consult your doctor about either adding, or switching to, a more conventional antidepressant. On the other hand, if you have detected a partial response and your symptoms are not too severe, you may want to wait a further few weeks before deciding on making any other medical changes.

3. Suggestions for Those Who Fall Somewhere in Between Feeling Mildly Blue and Suffering from Major Clinical Depression

Technically, those who don't quite meet diagnoses of major depressive disorder or dysthymia are known as subsyndromal. Studies on subsyndromal conditions have found that they can actually be quite disabling, often causing as much misery and costing those suffering from them as many days off work as the full-blown syndromes themselves. Clearly this is a midzone where judgment is required as to whether to involve a doctor or not. It's not a cold, it's not pneumonia, it's more like bronchitis or laryngitis, something nasty but not deadly. Seeking out medical attention is certainly the prudent course in such situations, but in reality, concerns about finances and other considerations frequently cause people to take matters into their own hands. Whether or not you choose to involve a physician in the treatment of your symptoms, St. John's wort can certainly be used, often to good effect. Follow the same guidelines for dosing and monitoring as outlined above.

4. Recommendations for Those with Severe Depression

If your depression is severe, I recommend that you start treatment with a conventional antidepressant as opposed to St. John's wort.

I would regard depression as being severe if it disrupts important functions, such as personal relationships or work, to a major degree, if it is seriously interfering with physical functions such as sleeping or eating, or if it is accompanied by a sense of hopelessness or suicidal ideas or plans. To date, there has been only one study with St. John's wort for relatively severe depression. Although the results of that study revealed a beneficial effect of St. John's wort, approximately equivalent to a modest dose of a conventional antidepressant, there are numerous studies indicating the value of more conventional antidepressants in severe depression. At this point the benefits of St. John's wort for severe depression must be considered somewhat experimental and a more proven first-line approach makes more sense, given how much is at stake when depressive symptoms are severe. Severe depression can jeopardize a person's job, relationship, or the successful outcome of a project. Of even greater concern is the danger of suicide, which is a major risk in severe depression. A delay resulting from starting with a less well established approach is therefore too risky. A doctor should be consulted and a trial of a conventional antidepressant should be initiated without delay.

If You Are Already on One or More Antidepressants or Mood-Regulating Drugs and Are Considering Either Switching to St. John's Wort or Adding It to Your Current Regimen, It Is Worth Asking Yourself These Questions

> Is my current regimen controlling my depressive symptoms with an acceptably low level of side effects, am I still depressed (at least in part), or am I bothered by unacceptable side effects?

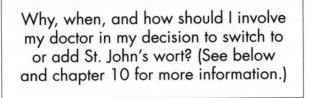

Why, when, and how should I involve
my doctor in my decision to switch to
or add St. John's wort? (See below
and chapter 10 for more information.)

How should I go about switching to St.
John's wort or adding it to my current
regimen? (See below and chapter 12
for more information.)

How can I monitor my progress on the
new regimen? (See above.)

Where can I find out more about how
to use St. John's wort, including when
it is combined with other medications?
(See below as well as chapter 12.)

If you are currently being treated with one or more anti-depressants and are considering using St. John's wort, you need to ask how to proceed if:

1. You are doing well, your depressive symptoms are under good control, and side effects are at an acceptably low level.

2. You are already being treated for depression but are not doing as well as you would like either because your depressive symptoms are not under control or because side effects are unacceptable or undesirable.

1. Suggestions for Those Who Are Doing Well, Whose Depressive Symptoms Are Under Good Control, and Where Side Effects Are At an Acceptably Low Level

I recommend that you stick with your existing program. If your depression is well controlled and the side effects of your current treatment regimen are acceptable, you have reason to be thankful. Not everyone attains such a good resolution for the problem of depression. Don't switch to St. John's wort just because it is an herbal remedy or an exciting form of treatment. It might be less beneficial than what you are already taking and you might experience a relapse of your symptoms. It is more important to feel better than to be fashionable. So don't mess with success, and enjoy your good health.

2. Suggestions for Those Who Are Already Being Treated for Depression but Are Not Doing As Well As They Would Like to Either Because Their Depressive Symptoms Are Not Under Control or Because Side Effects Are Unacceptable or Undesirable

If your depression has been treated with only partial success and the side effects of your current treatment are acceptable, it may be worth adding St. John's wort to your current treatment regimen provided you are not being treated with the MAOI type of antidepressant. Brand names of MAOI antidepressants are Nardil and Parnate, and if you are taking them, your doctor should have warned you not to eat cheese or drink red wine while on these medications. Apart from the MAOIs, it appears that St. John's wort can be combined with all other antidepressants quite safely, provided this is done under medical supervision.

Be sure to consult your doctor before adding St. John's wort to what you are already taking. Even though the herbal remedy is available over the counter and is regarded as a nutritional supplement, it is an active antidepressant and can interact with the medications your doctor has already prescribed. That is, after all, the very reason for adding it in the first place. As such, it cannot be considered in the same category as adding vitamin C to your existing medications, which would not necessitate a call to your doctor.

Suggested Dosing Schedule

Since you are already taking an antidepressant, it is wise to start St. John's wort more slowly than if there were no other antidepressant in the picture. Start with one 300-mg tablet (or even a 150-mg tablet) for at least a week before adding the second tablet, then wait a second week before adding the third tablet. You may once again need to wait at least four weeks before being able to judge with any degree of confidence whether the addition of the herb has made a difference in your mood. In some cases, however, evidence of mood improvement can be detected much sooner. Side effects may also develop more readily, and I have encountered jitteriness, muscle twitches, confusion, and hypomanic symptoms in a few of my patients in whom the herbal remedy was added to Prozac. If such symptoms occur, be sure to report them to your doctor without delay. They may signify too much serotonin in the brain, resulting in the so-called serotonin syndrome, which I describe in more detail on pages 183–185.

If you are currently being treated with conventional antidepressants and are experiencing unacceptable side effects, you will need to reduce the dosage of antidepressants that you are currently taking before getting relief from these side effects. In other words, simply adding St. John's wort is not going to remove the side effects caused by another antidepressant. After decreasing the dose of the other medication, you can then add St. John's wort in the hope that it will have the beneficial effects of the drug that is being tapered without its adverse effects. I usually recommend overlapping the two drugs and moving slowly in reducing the dosage of the old one while increasing the dosage of the new one. That strategy is often used in switching from one antidepressant to another and tends to minimize the unpleasant feelings that may be associated with the medication shifts. Once again, listen to what your body is telling you, as it is often the best guide as to how to pace the medication changes. All the same reasons for involving your doctor in this change of medications apply here as much as in the previous example or, possibly, more so. When you reduce an antidepressant that has been working, you risk suffering a relapse and may really need your doctor's help and support in getting the medication adjustment right and helping you get through the transition period.

In summary, if you are considering starting St. John's wort to treat depressive symptoms, develop a game plan, which should involve all of the following elements:

- Decide where your symptoms fit in on the depressive spectrum, which can range from mild to very severe.

- Decide whether it makes sense to involve a doctor in your treatment.

- If you decide to take St. John's wort, review the guidelines for how to start treatment, adjust dosage, and monitor response.

While all of these elements have been discussed to some degree in this chapter in order to provide you with an overall approach to treatment, much more detail is provided elsewhere in the book, which should answer many, if not all, of the questions you may have about St. John's wort and how best to use it.

10

WHEN, WHY, AND HOW TO INVOLVE A DOCTOR IN THE TREATMENT OF YOUR DEPRESSION

In earlier chapters I provided some guidelines as to how to diagnose your own depression and when it might make sense to involve a doctor in its treatment. In this chapter, I go into greater detail about this. Essentially, there are five reasons for involving a doctor in the treatment of depression. First, if depression is severe, it is both costly and risky to treat it on your own. In addition, there is far less evidence for the efficacy of St. John's wort in severe depression than there is for more conventional antidepressants. Second, other conditions may masquerade as depression. A visit to a doctor may uncover another reason for symptoms and lead to a different type of treatment for them. Treating such conditions with conventional antidepressant strategies may be ineffective and will delay the treatment of the underlying problem. Third, there may be other psychiatric problems that are worthy of attention in their own right and depression may even be secondary to these other problems. Treating these other conditions may be the first order of business and requires the help of a physician. Fourth, it can be difficult to be the best judge of your own mood and progress and a skillful observer and experienced clinician is an invaluable companion in the treatment of depression. Finally, depression is a lonely condition and a good doctor is also like a good friend who cheers you on through the dark wood into a better and brighter place.

1. Severe Depression Needs Urgent Medical Attention

The voice on my answering machine says, "I am calling to cancel my appointment for tomorrow. I am just too upset to come in and talk about it." This is the paradox of severe depression. It is a downward spiral. You feel so bad you have no wish to seek assistance nor any hope that it will help. You become more isolated and depressed. Work and relationships suffer, compounding the problem, and so it goes. You can be helped but you have to get to the doctor if that is to happen. And sometimes, if you can't manage to do so yourself, a loved one or friend must take you there. Often, this takes relatively little work on the friend's part, but what a difference it can make!

Someone calls to ask me to see his friend, who is very depressed and needs help immediately. I am closed to new referrals I say, but something in the friend's voice changes my mind. If someone has a friend who cares so much for him, somehow that makes me care more too. I become involved, recruited to be a member of the team and help the friend out of his depression. Two months later the friend is completely well (on Zoloft, incidentally, not St. John's wort). It was too acute and serious to warrant my trying the herbal antidepressant, though in future, as we learn more about the herb, it may become a first-line treatment even for more serious depression.

Serious depression can cost a person his or her life. It can wreak havoc with relationships and jobs. It is a medical emergency—and it is treatable. So it is clearly a reason to seek out medical help without delay. And if you have a friend or loved one who is severely depressed, do go the extra mile or two to connect him or her with a good doctor. It is really worth the trouble and effort to do so.

2. Other Conditions Can Masquerade As Depression

Some of the symptoms of depression may be the result of a different condition. Low energy level and fatigue may be symptoms of a medical condition, such as low thyroid functioning, which can be diagnosed easily by means of a simple blood test. But there are other conditions as well that can masquerade as depression.

A neighbor of mine, a highly successful scientist and a charming person in his midfifties, seemed to undergo a change of personality over the course of about a year. During this time, he walked around feeling fatigued and down in the dumps for many months. His sleep was restless and he would frequently wake up during the night. These symptoms might easily have been mistaken for depression. A visit to his doctor and, subsequently, to a sleep laboratory, however, revealed that he had a relatively common condition known as sleep apnea. He stopped breathing for short intervals numerous times during the course of the night, which would wake him up. As a result of his breathing difficulties, his brain was not receiving sufficient oxygen. Small wonder that he was exhausted during the day, felt miserable, and had difficulty concentrating. He was sleep deprived and his brain was short of oxygen. The problem was entirely corrected by a continuous positive air pressure (CPAP) machine, which ensures that he receives sufficient oxygen throughout the night. He became his cheerful self once more and I would see him tirelessly mowing his lawn and attending to his yard. We would once again chat and share jokes, and his mood was completely restored with the help of one critical substance upon which all of our lives depend—oxygen.

This same person later developed weakness and tiredness and again lost his usual ability to concentrate and function normally. Another visit to the doctor and some simple blood tests revealed that his blood chemistry was abnormal. This turned out to be due to a rare tumor of the adrenal gland. Removal of the tumor corrected the problem and restored him once again to his previous high level of functioning.

In summary, many of the symptoms of depression are not unique to this condition, but may also be the result of medical conditions, some of which, such as low thyroid levels or sleep apnea, are relatively common while others, such as tumors of the adrenal, are rather rare. A visit to a competent physician can often help sort out whether there may be a medical condition masquerading as depression. Even if at first you choose not to go to a physician but decide instead to try and treat your own depression, it is still worth bearing these other medical conditions in mind in case the symptoms do not resolve within a reasonable amount of time.

3. Depression May Coexist With, or Be Secondary To, Another Psychiatric Condition

Sometimes one type of psychiatric condition can mimic another. For example, an accountant in his midforties was referred to me for treatment of his low mood. He was very discouraged about his work, where he was constantly in trouble for procrastinating. He was very intelligent and had no difficulty understanding the complexities of his clients' finances, but somehow he had insurmountable problems with deadlines. He would leave things till the last minute when, by staying up all night working crazily, he would almost always succeed in getting the work done on time. But these last-minute all-nighters were becoming tiresome not only to my patient but to his associates as well. As a consequence, he was under pressure to work in a more steady and even manner and he was depressed at his difficulty in doing so.

Careful questioning revealed that he had suffered from attentional difficulties since childhood, had never performed up to his potential, and had always relied upon the intense pressure of deadlines and the prospects of failure to motivate himself to get anything done. In lectures and classes, he would lose track of what the lecturer or teacher was saying. He was extremely distractable and often left tasks—particularly boring and unpleasant ones such as paperwork—half completed as his attention shifted to something which at that moment he found more interesting. I diagnosed him as suffering from attention deficit disorder (ADD), prescribed Ritalin, a stimulant, and recommended certain behavioral changes in the way he approached his work. His work habits improved swiftly and dramatically and he soon felt much more cheerful. He turned out to be someone whose depressed mood was the result of another problem, the attention deficit disorder, which responded to treatments that are specifically helpful for that condition. An antidepressant alone would have been unlikely to correct his fundamental problem, namely, his attentional difficulties.

Even if a person is indeed depressed, it is worth going to see a doctor to determine whether some other treatable condition may be present in addition to the depression. Shakespeare noted that "when sorrows come, they come not as single spies but in battalions." And so it is that depression is often accompanied by some other condition, such as a drug or alcohol problem, attention deficit disorder, or an eating disorder. If these conditions are present, they deserve to be handled in their own right with the appropriate treatment. People with more than one condition often require more than one type of treatment to get the best results.

4. It Is Hard to Be the Best Judge and Manager of Your Own Moods

When you are depressed it is easy to lose your objectivity. Often it seems as though your unhappy feelings are a reasonable response to the behavior of others, whereas it may be that others are withdrawing from you because of your depression. Similarly, a setback at work may be the result of poor concentration and the inability to focus, which are well-known symptoms of depression. A good clinician will point these facts out to you and prescribe medications or suggest other types of treatment so as to control depressive symptoms that have been only partially treated. One useful way to monitor your own moods is to keep a log of them, such as the one provided on pages 217–218. Learning to evaluate your level of depression is an acquired art, and after being in treatment with a good clinician for some time, many people become extremely skillful at gauging and managing their own moods.

5. A Doctor As a Companion

In a recent article, the eminent physician and author Sherwin Nuland writes about the deficiencies of modern medicine, in which the doctor treats the disease but not the patient who suffers from it. Being ill is a lonely and scary condition; of all illnesses, depression must surely be one of the loneliest and scariest. A good doctor should be a source of comfort to you in your illness and in the recovery process. You would do well to invest the time and energy in finding a doctor who is not only technically competent but is also able to play this critical role.

Choosing a Doctor

I can't emphasize enough how important is the choice of a doctor. I am often astonished by how some highly discriminating people, who are careful in the selection of their barber or hairdresser, and will go to great lengths to buy the right car at the right price, will take potluck with whatever doctor is assigned to them by their health maintenance organization. I always suggest that people go to doctors recommended by other doctors, figuring that if you're in the trade yourself, you know the wheat from the chaff.

Credentials are of some value in choosing a good doctor, but sometimes doctors trained at the best places can also be conceited and closed to new ideas. In seeking a doctor, find someone who is smart, up to date, sympathetic, open-minded, and not too impressed with his or her own opinions—someone who you feel listens to you and really hears what you're saying. Finally, keep an eye on your doctor. Even the best doctors are only human; they can make mistakes and don't always think of all the possibilities. Even if you are in treatment with a good doctor, you still have some responsibility to use your wits to be sure that you get the best possible care.

Extricating Yourself from an Unsuitable Doctor

A good doctor should not only keep up with the literature but should also be open to learning new things. Ignorance is human and often forgivable; it is, after all, a treatable condition. Closed-mindedness, however, is hard to fix; if your doctor is not open to new information, that is a real problem, since medicine is constantly changing and new diagnostic and treatment approaches are regularly being developed. It can also be very distressing to end up with a doctor who, rightly or wrongly, reflexively dismisses your point of view, as illustrated by the following cautionary tale.

Jennifer, a woman of about forty, has suffered for some years from both winter depressions and attention deficit disorder (ADD). I have treated her with Prozac, accompanied by light therapy for her winter depressions and with Ritalin year-round for her ADD. She is an intelligent and artistic person who has used her sensitivity to light to create paintings in which bright colors sweep across large sheets of canvas, giving the impression of vivid sunsets or tropical birds flying across azure skies.

Troubled by the weight gain that she has experienced since starting Prozac, Jennifer went to see her internist, who was listed in a local magazine as one of the best in the area. She explained to him that the weight gain appeared to be a direct result of being on Prozac. He told her that that was impossible, that Prozac causes weight loss, not weight gain. She told him that I had mentioned that I had seen weight gain as a result of Prozac and related antidepressant medications and that this may follow an initial period of weight loss. She pointed out that I had even made mention of this observation in a book of mine. He told her she must have misunderstood me and was certainly mistaken in her facts. She began to cry. He became increasingly upset with her for disagreeing with him and ended up actually discharging her from his practice. Although the experience was quite traumatic for Jennifer, she is obviously better off without this doctor. The moral of the story is simple. If a doctor is unwilling to listen to you and take your comments seriously, you are better off with someone else. All of us should have our minds open to new information.

Another patient of mine did not wait for her doctor to fire her. She fired him. This woman in her early twenties had suffered from recurrent depressions for many years. She had been treated with Zoloft with some success, but at therapeutic dosages felt uncomfortably "wired." She decreased the dosage of Zoloft and wanted to add St. John's wort to the mix but her doctor, having read that the herb should not be mixed with other antidepressants, told her that it was dangerous to do so. The young woman searched the literature, found new reports contradicting the early warnings that her doctor had read, and decided to try St. John's wort on her own in conjunction with Zoloft. She responded very well to the combination and experienced no side effects whatsoever. She continued to see her doctor regularly and, after some time, plucked up the courage to tell him what she had done. He became very angry and chastised her for taking the herbal remedy behind his back. At that point she decided to change doctors. She could forgive him for not being aware of the latest information about the herb and for his tendency to be controlling, but it really hurt her to think that he would be more upset that she had defied him rather than happy that she was feeling better.

Sometimes it is as important to extricate yourself from an unsuitable doctor as it is to find a suitable one.

11

MAKING ST. JOHN'S WORT PART OF AN ANTIDEPRESSANT LIFESTYLE

Live in rooms full of light.
Avoid heavy foods.
Be moderate in the drinking of wine.
Take massage, baths, exercise, and gymnastics.
Fight insomnia with gentle rocking or the sound
    of running water.
Change surroundings and take long journeys.
Strictly avoid frightening ideas.
Indulge in cheerful conversation and amusements.
Listen to music.

—A. CORNELIUS CELSUS, "ADVICE TO
MELANCHOLICS," FIRST CENTURY A.D.

It is typical for us humans to expect everything to fly into
our mouths without work, art, effort, grief and suffering.
But all of this is not God's way; rather, it is His will that
we should work hard for our food and that we should
want to support both ourselves and those around us.

—PARACELSUS, 1493–1541,
COLLECTED WRITINGS

There is an old joke about a bookseller who is trying to sell a book to a student. "It will do half your work for you," he claims. "Great," says the student. "I'll buy two copies." It is only human for us to want to have all our work done for us or all our problems solved by a simple remedy such as a pill. The bad news and, of course, it is not really new at all, is that wondrous though a pill may be—St. John's wort included—it will not cure all that ails you. The good news is that there are so many ways to help yourself, many of them quite painless and even pleasurable, as the advice of A. Cornelius Celsus above would suggest. Celsus was the physician to the emperor Tiberius, a cruel, powerful, and frightening man, and the gentleness of Celsus's advice was perhaps as much politic as it was wise. Paracelsus, an outspoken man, fearless and impolitic in the conduct of his own life, had no qualms about expressing himself frankly. According to him, if you wanted your life to be better, you needed to exert some effort to make it so.

There are merits to both men's points of view. In my own dealings with depressed people, I have found many ways in which modifying elements of one's life can contribute enormously to an antidepressant lifestyle that works beautifully in conjunction with antidepressant medications, including St. John's wort. In this chapter we will consider some of the many ways in which you can help take control of your life and conquer your own depression.

Become a Shrewd Observer of Your Own Moods

Just as you need to have some sense of the weather in order to know how to dress and whether to take a raincoat or an umbrella along, so you need to have a good sense of your mood in order to make the necessary adjustments to your lifestyle. Sometimes fluctuations in mood occur during a single day. A piece of bad news, a valuable object mislaid, or an encounter with an unpleasant person may plunge you into a gloomy frame of mind for several hours, only to be reversed later in the day by a piece of good news, the recovery of your lost treasure, or a visit with a friend. Recognizing the connection between your mood and these external events turns out to be enormously useful in making the hour-by-hour adjustments to help even out your mood throughout the day.

Other mood fluctuations occur over the course of days and are less easy to recognize. For example, people may become depressed a few days after the clocks are turned back at the end of autumn, after returning from abroad, or after a big party. In these three situations the deterioration in mood may be due, respectively, to the hour's decrease in afternoon daylight, jet lag, or the delayed effects of alcohol. One useful strategy for those who experience unexplained dips in mood is to keep a daily mood log, such as the one shown on pages 217–218, which will help you recognize the connection between mood fluctuations and external events. At times such logs can be crucial in convincing you that a clear pattern exists. For example, it was only after she had kept a log for several months that one of my patients was willing to concede that the alcohol she consumed on Saturday night was responsible for the dip in mood experienced two or three days later. Finally, there are mood changes that have a longer periodicity, such as the monthly mood changes caused by premenstrual syndrome or the annual mood fluctuations that occur with the change of the seasons in people with SAD or the winter blues.

Mood may change with the environment—physical, climatic, or human. One of my patients would feel depressed every time she went to her office. This seemed strange, as she liked her colleagues and was passionate about the work itself. The clues to her depression lay in her associated symptoms—headache, dizziness, fatigue, and difficulties with short-term memory. She worked in an airtight office building full of office chemicals—printer cartridges, copiers, fax machines, and other sources of organic solvents. She was a victim of the so-called sick-building syndrome and depression is one of the key symptoms that affect people suffering from that disorder. One patient with seasonal affective disorder experienced depression after she moved from a bright high-rise apartment to a dim basement studio. A third patient became depressed every time she visited her mother-in-law. The patient was very self-conscious about her looks and was constantly battling to lose weight. Somehow her mother-in-law always managed to direct the conversation to the patient's figure, often in the guise of a compliment. "That dress really suits you," she would say, "it's just right for your shape. Where did you find it?" This would invariably make the patient self-conscious and depressed. In all of these cases, the first step in handling the problem was understanding it. An old medical adage is that you cannot treat before you diagnose. I therefore recommend that if you are of a moody disposition, become your own diagnostician, find out what is depressing you, and then proceed to take remedial steps.

Taking Control of Your Life

Some of the most helpful things you can do to live an antidepressant lifestyle involve taking control of your life wherever possible. One well-known animal model of depression, developed by Martin Seligman, is learned helplessness. In this model, rats in cages are given electrical shocks at random until, presumably realizing that there is nothing they can do to prevent these shocks, they simply give up and lie down, resigned or, perhaps, depressed. Life may feel like that to some people. At work, you may be faced with one difficult situation after another. Your boss may be constantly disgruntled or repeatedly abusive. Similarly, in marriage, it sometimes feels as though you just can't win. No matter what you do or say, you end up in trouble with your spouse. These are topics of satire, but in reality they are not very funny. For example, in the highly successful British comedy series *Fawlty Towers*, the unfortunate innkeeper, Basil Fawlty, is always falling afoul of his wife. On one occasion she harangues him about his gambling. When, later in the episode, she checks on whether he has been betting on the horses again (which he has), he responds, "No, dear, that avenue of pleasure has been closed off to me." In depression, where avenues of pleasure are already closed off to the depressed person, it is particularly important that all sources of unhappiness be tackled or, where possible, avoided.

Tackling Stress

There are many ways of tackling or managing stress and mastering these techniques inevitably pays off by promoting an antidepressant lifestyle. Improving interpersonal skills, for example, is one way of reducing the feeling that others are a constant source of unavoidable and uncontrollable stress. When I first began to supervise research assistants, I would observe that they often seemed harried and anxious. On one occasion, as a result of a shuffling of government personnel, a senior manager was temporarily assigned to me as a research assistant. I delegated several tasks to him and after the first week of working under my direction, he asked to meet with me. He explained that the number of tasks I had assigned him were more than he was able to manage competently in the course of his working hours. Would I be good enough, he asked, to indicate to him my priorities so that if he was unable to complete all the tasks by the week's end, the least important task would remain undone. My research assistant had taught me two invaluable lessons. Not only did I learn to become a better manager, to set priorities and be more realistic about what could be accomplished in the time available, but I learned how someone who is subordinate in an organization can politely set limits and manage his or her level of daily stress.

If you are feeling under pressure at work, take some time to analyze the situation. Make a list of all the sources of stress and then try to figure out solutions to each of them. It is in the interest of the other parties involved to have these stresses resolved as well. Consider ways of presenting the problem to your boss, coworker, or even supervisee in such a way as to point out how it would be mutually beneficial if the stresses could be alleviated. For example, the final product might be superior, production might be more efficient, or the working environment more conducive to creativity or productivity. All of these goals can be legitimately presented as being in the interest of both workers and management.

Exactly the same principles apply in a marriage or other type of relationship, only more so. In these situations all parties involved usually have major investments at multiple, different levels. For example, in a marriage, it is in both parties' interests to get along, not only because it is more pleasant to do so, but also for the sake of mutual investments in the form of children and other common goals. Once again, sources of stress can be identified and communicated to your partner and if this is done in the right way, it can diminish levels of stress, relieve the tension in the relationship, and promote an antidepressant lifestyle. The key is always to present the situation as a shared issue that would benefit both individuals to solve together. Let us say, for example, that a husband comes home from work and goes straight to the fridge for a beer, in the process ignoring his wife. She is bound to feel neglected, angry, and perhaps depressed. At this point she has a choice. She can attack her husband for his callous and brutish behavior or she can take a more collaborative approach. Attacking him may make her feel better in the short run but is bound to make the problem worse. A collaborative approach may have a better chance of working in the long run. This could involve: (1) empathy—"I understand that you are stressed and tired at the end of a hard day"; (2) communication of her feelings—"I feel the same way after running after the kids all day"; (3) involving him in solving the problem—"Can you think of some way that we can unwind together"; and (4) demonstration of what's in it for him to do so—"so that we can support each other at difficult times and maybe even figure out a way of having some fun in the process?" Obviously, the way in which she chooses to handle the communication is likely to influence the outcome of the evening and either exacerbate or ameliorate her depression.

Part of the skill involved in such communications is picking the right time. A perceptive husband might recognize, for example, that the three days before his wife's period are not the best time to discuss the large charges she has run up on the credit card. Conversely, an insightful wife learns to discern her husband's moods and bides her time before discussing with him how she could use more help from him around the house or with the children.

It is also important to recognize that depression frequently causes stress in a relationship. This is, of course, an additional reason to treat the depression biologically. The partner of the depressed person often feels neglected. Feelings of depression can be contagious and there is a natural tendency to want to avoid a depressed person, which can isolate the person further and cause the depression to deepen.

There are some important pointers for the partner or family member of a depressed person to bear in mind.

- Don't take the depression personally. This is easier said than done, because it is easy to misinterpret a depressed person's silent withdrawal as hostility targeted against you. But remember, this is a cardinal symptom of depression—the person probably behaves that way toward everyone.

- It is not your responsibility to turn the depressed person's mood around. The depression is not your fault. Frequently, the family member feels responsible for the depressed person's mood, which makes him or her angry, since at times nothing seems to cheer up the depressed person. This can result in a tendency for friends and family members to give up on the depressed person and withdraw, which compounds the depressed person's sense of isolation. You can and should be supportive. It is particularly worth trying to help your friend or loved one get appropriate assistance. But you cannot expect to have a direct effect on the other person's mood. It is too much of a burden to place on yourself and is bound to leave you feeling resentful.

- Don't ignore the depressed person and enhance his or her sense of isolation. Do what you can to include the person in activities in a nondemanding way. For example, a husband might suggest going out to a restaurant for dinner with his wife, who may feel cheered up by the food, the setting, and the friendly attention. On the other hand, suggesting that it might cheer her up to have guests over is unlikely to have its intended beneficial effect because of the demands that suggestion will place on her to perform and be sociable, which might be the last things in the world that she feels like doing.

There is a great deal that a depressed person can do to keep his or her loved one involved even while in a depressed state.

- Simply acknowledging the depression and its impact can be helpful. For example, a wife is likely to respond favorably to her depressed husband if he says, "I know I have been down and not much fun lately, but I am trying to turn things around as best I can. Thanks for hanging in there with me." The partner of a depressed person becomes starved for any positive feedback and comments such as this are generally greatly appreciated.

- Even if you are feeling sad and withholding, as is often the case when one is depressed, it pays to make a point of expressing appreciation to your friend or loved one for gestures of kindness.

- It can also be useful to pinpoint specific things that your loved one can do that would make you feel better. This helps him or her to feel useful and counteracts the powerlessness typically experienced by those who surround and care about a depressed person.

So important are interpersonal skills in helping people overcome and avoid depression that an entire type of psychotherapy for depression, called "interpersonal therapy," has been developed around these principles.

There are many types of stress other than interpersonal difficulties that may confront a depressed person and make matters worse. These include physical illness, financial difficulties, and the loss of a loved one. For all these different types of situations, help can be obtained from different types of experts, for example, an empathic and competent physician, a financial adviser, or a religious or spiritual leader. A good doctor should not only provide specific help for symptoms but also comfort and reassurance. I have seen people in serious financial difficulty who have been greatly relieved after turning their affairs over to a debt counselor or obtaining help and guidance from a financial planner. And innumerable people have been comforted and supported over the centuries by their priests, ministers, or rabbis. Of course, caveat emptor applies whenever one turns to any guide or authority figure for help. Ultimately, you have to be the judge as to whether a so-called expert is helping you or not. As always, stay tuned to your mood barometer to judge the quality of assistance you are receiving.

Flight into Health

The two main ways in which all animals deal with stress are fight and flight. It is important to remember that a major way of managing stress is to leave it behind, to quit. The term "quitter" has a negative connotation in our culture, but sometimes quitting is the smartest thing you can do. "Take your job and shove it" are the words of a country-and-western song. Who has not considered such an approach at one time or another? Of course, it is generally unwise to quit one's job impulsively or without due reflection. But there are times when, after careful consideration, the healthiest thing to do may be to leave an unpleasant job and find some other form of employment.

Epidemiological studies have shown that depression is increasing in frequency in young people. One possible reason for this increase may be the escalating stress placed on workers in modern organizations, where competition may be greater and job security and working conditions less appealing than in earlier decades. The cartoon strip *Dilbert* has been enormously successful, in large measure because it accurately captures and parodies the stressful and depersonalizing atmosphere of the modern workplace. In many organizations, people are being expected to work harder for smaller rewards and with less control over their work environment. This can be extremely demoralizing. To address some of these problems, many people have attempted to gain greater control over their working environment by quitting their jobs and working as freelancers. Although in doing so they have sometimes had to take a cut in pay, many have found that the greater control they have over their lives more than compensates for this sacrifice. They enjoy setting their own hours, choosing their work, and, best of all, not having a boss and a bureaucracy to answer to. If you are feeling disempowered at work, it may be worth considering whether working for yourself might be preferable.

I want to sound one major cautionary note, however. If you are in the midst of a bad depression, it is unwise to make any major life decision until the worst of the depression is behind you. When you are depressed, everything seems bad, including your job. I have encountered people who have quit their jobs in the midst of a profound depression and then regretted it later, after they felt better, at which time they may have come to appreciate the more positive aspects of their former work. The best approach in such situations is first, to treat the depression medically, for example, with St. John's wort or some other antidepressant, and after you are feeling a great deal better, to consider the possibility that an unpleasant job situation may put you at risk for further depression or may hinder your complete recovery.

Just as it can be helpful to quit a bad job, so it can be healthy to leave a bad relationship. When this is a relationship of major significance, like a marriage, it is obviously worth spending a good deal of time and energy in making the decision as to whether to stay and try to work things out or to move on. Sometimes the most exciting relationships are also those that are most likely to trigger depressions. Dr. Donald Klein described a condition that he called "hysteroid dysphoria" in which the affected person, usually but not invariably a woman, easily becomes enmeshed in a series of romantic relationships, each of which takes on the same pattern. Initially there is an intense feeling of falling in love, associated with enormous passion and elation. This is invariably followed by rejection or disappointment as the object of the woman's affections either rejects her or no longer appears to be a prince on a white horse after all but rather, in the eyes of the angry and disappointed lover, the horse's rear end. A crashing depression ensues that is relieved only by the arrival of the next prince. While medications often help with such problems, making someone less vulnerable to being swept off her feet and then dropped unceremoniously, it is obviously critical to address the underlying issue as well. The affected person is looking to her lover as a means of regulating her mood; until she learns how to stop doing so, she is destined to suffer from recurrent depressions as a consequence. Psychotherapy and social support can help in this process. Even more valuable than getting out of toxic relationships is learning how to avoid getting into them in the first place. Often, the resolution involves entering a relationship with a different type of person, someone who is perhaps less thrilling than previous partners but who is a more dependable and ultimately a more satisfying mate.

In the days when psychoanalysis was the dominant force in psychiatry, the idea of improving your mood by leaving a problem behind was often frowned upon and referred to somewhat pejoratively as a flight into health. The idea was that you needed to work on a problem to resolve it rather than run away from it. Of course, it often makes sense to work on problems, as I have mentioned, but let us not underestimate the value of leaving a problem behind. It is, after all, a basic animal instinct to run from certain threats and a principle of environmental medicine to recognize toxic influences and avoid them. There is no reason why that same good sense should not apply to the treatment of depression as well.

Social Supports

Even more important than experts in alleviating the stresses of everyday lives are our family and friends—our everyday supports. Researchers have found that even in rat models of depression, social supports play a crucial role in mediating the effects of stress on the development of depressive-type symptoms. In one model, researchers introduce a dominant rat to a more submissive rat alone in a cage. The dominant rat will attack the submissive one and beat it into a state of submission, which the researchers have suggested is the equivalent of a depressed state. If they then place the submissive rat alone in another cage, it will remain in a cowering, submissive posture. This will not occur if the rat is returned to a cage with its littermates. The presence of these other rats appears to provide relief from the depressive symptoms, which do not persist.

Although it may be novel to consider the importance of social supports in protecting against depression in other species, its value in shoring up the human spirit should come as no surprise. In small communities all over the world, there is considerable support from neighbors, friends, and family in times of need. A good friend or, better still, a circle of friends is one of the best nonpharmacological antidepressants you can find. Cicero, writing about friendship about two thousand years ago, observed that a joy is doubled and a sorrow halved when it is shared with a friend.

In our modern industrial society, however, where people move around more frequently and often live in more impersonal settings, the support of family and friends is often lacking. This is reflected in the Beatles' famous song "Eleanor Rigby," where the group sings about all the lonely people and asks where they all belong. Eleanor Rigby, the lonely person who picks up the rice in the church where the wedding has been, is a symbol of those of us who are detached from a group of supportive people. Where do such people belong? Where can they find comfort and support in times of need? Others who fall into this category are those who come from dysfunctional families, which appear to be ever increasing in prevalence. Often, such people feel that they cannot turn to their families in times of need because they will not be understood and accepted for who they are. Such people can find enormous support and comfort by turning to support or recovery groups.

Support and Recovery Groups: The Best Deal in Town

Support groups now exist for many serious and debilitating illnesses, and depression is no exception in this regard. Such organizations may provide:

- up-to-date information about a specific condition

- meetings to help members and their families cope with depression

- peer counseling

- formal recovery programs

A listing of available support groups that deal with depression and related disorders is provided in the resource section at the end of this book.

Recovery, or twelve-step, groups are modeled on the principles set down by Alcoholics Anonymous, which was the first such group to be developed. There are currently recovery groups for drug addicts, sex and love addicts, compulsive gamblers, overeaters, and adult children of alcoholics. There are also separate groups for the spouses, partners, or family members of those who participate in these various groups. Recovery groups combine a program consisting of working through a series of specific steps, with fellowship, support, and simple wisdom. In meetings, people learn that they are not alone in their unhappiness. They are encouraged to talk freely and are listened to in a nonjudgmental way without being challenged or confronted. There is a spirit of respect for what people have to say and the problems they are grappling with.

I have encouraged many of my patients with addictions (with or without depression) to go to an appropriate recovery group, often with good results. At times I have managed to locate another group member who is willing to pick the newcomer up and take him or her to a meeting of the group. I have encountered considerable reluctance in my patients to go along with this suggestion and they have frequently cited concerns about confidentiality and their professional reputations. Nevertheless, all those who have followed my suggestion have found such groups to be quite valuable. It is very important in choosing a group to pick one in which the other members come from a socioeconomic class similar to your own so that you can more easily identify with the other group members. Token contributions are requested of members. I often appeal to the ordinary human instinct (possibly genetically programmed) for finding a bargain by pointing out to my patients that at a dollar a meeting, recovery groups are the best deal in town.

Surprisingly, even some individuals who are not addicts have found that recovery groups can be helpful, and given the large number of groups available, it is usually not difficult to find one where one can feel at home. One of my patients, a woman in her midsixties, has suffered from severe intermittent depressions for decades despite my best efforts at medicating her with multiple antidepressants, including St. John's wort. She would qualify as an adult child of an alcoholic, as her mother was drunk through much of her childhood and died of cirrhosis of the liver when the patient was a young girl. She was reluctant, however, to go to a recovery group so I told her some of the slogans that members of recovery groups often repeat to themselves and to others by way of encouragement.

To my surprise, this extremely sophisticated woman, a veteran of many years of all sorts of psychotherapy, repeated the slogans to herself several times and wrote them down carefully. The slogans I shared with her were:

One day at a time.

Just get your body there; the rest will follow.

Fake it till you make it.

These are all useful slogans for the depressed person, who amplifies his or her troubles and projects them into the distant future. Take one day at a time, the first slogan urges. If you consider all possible future problems at once, they will seem overwhelming and you can drown in a sea of sorrows. In the case of an addict, this can drive the person to drink, use drugs, or act out in some addictive way. In a depressive person, it can drive him or her to despair. In contemplating some professional or social commitment, a depressed person frequently asks, "How can I possibly handle it?" Just get there, urges the second slogan. Often, your automatic pilot will take over and see you through. In a song written to encourage those in despair, the singer Billy Joel counsels the listener not to forget his second wind but rather to wait for the momentum to kick in. The woman mentioned above used this way of thinking to help her get to a wedding that she had no wish to attend. Once there, however, she surprised herself by having quite a good time and afterward felt very pleased that she had been able to come through for her friends and family. The slogan "Fake it till you make it" suggests that if you pretend you are managing, you might be surprised to discover that you really *are* managing after all. Things may turn out this way for all sorts of reasons. First, the anticipation of the task or event may be worse than the thing itself. In certain types of depression, it is impossible to anticipate pleasure, but once placed in a potentially pleasurable situation, you may actually be capable of enjoying it. Another reason for why you might make it after you fake it is related to daily or circadian rhythms of mood, whereby it is common for a person's depression to be at its worst in the morning and to improve as the day wears on.

Some people balk at recovery groups because many of the steps are geared around the concept of a Higher Power and, as such, may offend a person's religious sentiments or lack thereof. Nevertheless, the whole matter is generally handled with a light touch and in a noncoercive way that many people find acceptable.

In summary, support groups offer invaluable information and encouragement around specific illnesses, including depression, while recovery groups provide fellowship, wisdom, and tangible assistance for people with all manner of sorrows and problems.

Watching Your Alcohol Intake

Even if you don't have a defined problem with alcohol, it is very important for a person who suffers from depression to pay careful attention to your alcohol intake. First of all, alcohol is capable of interacting negatively with any drug that affects brain functioning. Even though one study of individuals taking St. John's wort suggested that the effect of alcohol on their coordination and ability to concentrate was no different from that seen in people on a placebo, I would recommend moderation in alcohol consumption to someone on St. John's wort just as I would to a person on any other type of antidepressant. In practical terms, this generally means no more than one glass of wine or a single shot of liquor (or at the most two), depending on an individual's tolerance. As always, it is important to exercise judgment when driving or operating machinery under such combined drug influences.

Even in those who appear to handle their alcohol very well in the hours after drinking it, I have often noticed a ripple effect on mood in the days that follow. This sometimes occurs after a very small amount of alcohol (even a single glass of wine) and takes the patient quite by surprise when the association is finally recognized. As I mentioned, sometimes it is only by logging one's mood on a daily basis that a person will come to appreciate that there is indeed a cause-and-effect relationship between drinking alcohol and becoming depressed.

The Benefits of Exercise—Even a Little

After treating hundreds of depressed people, I have become increasingly impressed with the value of exercise as an antidepressant. Conversely, I have often found that if a regular exerciser who is vulnerable to depression should become unable to exercise for any reason, depression frequently ensues. I know that it is a pain in the neck to be advised to exercise when you are depressed, and it may be the last thing in the world that you feel like doing. But it really works.

There are by now several controlled studies indicating the benefits of exercise in depression. All studies agree that exercise is superior to no treatment at all. Two studies found that combining exercise with counseling was superior to counseling alone. This bears out my experience that it pays to combine different forms of treatment in your efforts to overcome depression. Even exercise of low intensity can be beneficial, though some find that more vigorous aerobic sessions on a regular basis work better for them.

I am often told, "If I were able to motivate myself to exercise, I would not be depressed and wouldn't need it in the first place." I recommend that people do whatever it takes to make exercise workable and even pleasant. Sometimes this means finding a friend or workout buddy; sometimes it means hiring a trainer. Even though I am not generally depressed, I hire a trainer to help me adhere to a regular exercise program. If I know I have an appointment with someone at a certain time, I am much more likely to take my exercise seriously and not find some wonderful excuse to skip my exercise routine "just this once." In addition, a good trainer helps you pace yourself so as to maximize your gains while minimizing the likelihood of physical injuries.

Use your creativity in designing an exercise routine in a setting that works for you. One of my patients, for example, works out on a ski machine alongside her husband while watching videotaped movies. A friend jogs on a trampoline while listening to a prerecorded cassette of Baroque music that has a tempo that matches her jogging speed. Dance of all kinds can be appealing because of the combination of music, aerobic exercise, and companionship. But we differ from one another in taste and the key is to find what type of exercise works for you.

An important point to remember when beginning an exercise program is not to overdo it. An excellent way to sabotage a long-term exercise program is to injure your ankle or knee, which will put you out of commission for several weeks. This will, of course, be counterproductive and you might find yourself sympathizing with the words of Winston Churchill, who defended his lack of exercise by noting that he got enough exercise acting as pallbearer at the funerals of friends who exercised regularly. Depressed people are often careless about their physical health. So please remember to start slowly and carefully; if you do this, your exercise program will be much more rewarding over time.

Controlling Your Mood with Sleep

There is ample evidence that the amount and timing of your sleep can have a profound effect on your mood, and you can use this known relationship to your advantage. Once again, a log of your mood and sleep (see pages 217–218) may provide clues as to what the relationship might be. For example, you might note that after a few late nights, your depression is worse for the next several days. If so, an obvious solution will present itself to you—be sure to get to bed on time as regularly as possible and get sufficient sleep. In general, regular patterns of sleeping and waking, known in the trade as "good sleep hygiene," tend to promote more even mood control.

But the relationship between sleep and mood is not always so obvious. In the 1970s, Dr. Thomas Wehr and colleagues, working from a theory that a fundamental problem in depressed people was that the timing of their sleep was too late in relation to their other body rhythms, devised an antidepressant treatment called "phase advance of sleep." These researchers showed that if you move the onset and offset of sleep several hours earlier, in some depressed patients, for example, to five P.M. through one A.M., a remarkable improvement in mood will result within several days. Although this finding was of theoretical interest, it was regarded as impractical largely because people were unwilling to go to sleep and wake up at such inconvenient hours. Another curious relationship between sleep and depression, discovered even earlier than the phase advance treatment, is that in a depressed patient, a night of sleep deprivation is often followed by a remarkable improvement in mood on the following day. This counterintuitive effect was discovered accidentally by a depressed German woman, who observed that her mood was much better on the day following an all-night bicycle ride. Sleep deprivation has been disappointing as a treatment for depression because its benefits are generally rather short-lived, dissipating the very next day after a night of recovery sleep.

Recently Dr. Mathias Berger and colleagues in Germany have developed an ingenious way of combining sleep deprivation and phase advance of sleep so that the combined treatment is both effective and practical. In controlled studies they have deprived depressed patients of sleep for a single night and followed that with a regimen of phase-advanced sleep for several nights afterward. After achieving an antidepressant response, the researchers then moved the timing of sleep progressively later, an hour per night, over the next six days until they reached the patient's accustomed times of sleep onset and waking. Remarkably, without any medications whatsoever, these researchers obtained stable antidepressant responses in a high percentage of their patients. Although I have not as yet used this new combined sleep modification therapy in my own clinical practice, I am waiting for an opportunity to do so. Once again, a valuable antidepressant treatment is being developed in Germany and we would be well advised to pay attention to it sooner rather than later.

Live in Rooms Full of Light

In the chapter on seasonal affective disorder (SAD), I discussed the value of light therapy for those who become depressed during the dark days, whether these occur during the winter or at other times of the year. What is less well known, however, is that there is growing evidence that light therapy may also be beneficial for patients whose depressions are *not* seasonal or specifically related to environmental light at all. These people may benefit from enhanced environmental lighting by itself or, more commonly, in conjunction with other forms of antidepressant treatment.

Dr. Joachim Fisch and colleagues in Germany set out to investigate whether light therapy might enhance the response of depressed patients to treatment with St. John's wort. They divided forty depressed patients whose mood changes bore no specific relationship to the changing seasons into two groups of twenty each. Both groups received standard doses of hypericum—900 mg per day. In addition to this, one group was exposed to bright environmental light and the other to dim environmental light for two hours each day. They found that the group exposed to bright light showed superior antidepressant effects after two and four weeks of treatment. After six weeks, however, both groups fared equally well. They concluded that light therapy may speed up the antidepressant response to hypericum. Even if enhanced environmental lighting did no more than this, it would still be worth considering, since the weeks before an antidepressant kicks in may seem interminable to a person suffering from the painful symptoms of depression. It is especially difficult to keep up one's spirits and optimism during the early weeks of treatment, since there is no guarantee that the medications will actually work. Signs of an early response are therefore particularly welcome.

It is possible that enhancing environmental lighting may do more than simply speed up the response to an antidepressant—it may actually enhance the response. Although this effect has not yet been demonstrated for St. John's wort, Dr. Kasper and colleagues studied a group of depressed patients who had failed to respond to an adequate trial of Prozac. These researchers treated half of their patients with bright light and half with dim light while keeping them on Prozac. After two weeks, the patients receiving bright light showed significantly greater improvements than those receiving dim light treatment, an advantage that increased over the following two weeks of the study.

These studies suggest that combining bright light therapy with antidepressant medications, including St. John's wort, may be a valuable strategy for enhancing the speed and magnitude of the therapeutic response even in those depressed patients who have not suffered exclusively from winter depressions.

The known interaction between light and hypericum has raised concerns about possible harmful effects to the eyes in people receiving light therapy while on St. John's wort. So far, the only study that has addressed this question directly is that of Dr. Kasper and colleagues, who examined the eyes of their patients after two weeks of such combination therapy and found no eye changes. A recent study by Dr. Brockmöller and colleagues, showing very little increase in skin tanning in patients on clinically relevant doses of hypericum, is also encouraging in relation to the safety of combining St. John's wort and light therapy. Nevertheless, if you experience any eye irritation while on the combination, check with your doctor about it. What I recommend for my patients if they experience eye strain or irritation while receiving light therapy is that they try to decrease their exposure to bright light either by shortening the daily duration of treatment or sitting farther away from the light source until their eyes feel comfortable.

> Warning: If you have any history of eye problems, you should always consult an eye doctor before undertaking light therapy.

As the quote from A. Cornelius Celsus suggests, it is possible to derive benefits from enhanced environmental lighting without any formal therapy simply by brightening the interior of your house. This can be done with more lamps, including indirect lighting bounced off lightly colored surfaces. Bright colors, especially yellows and oranges, also seem to have a cheering effect on many of the light-sensitive people I have treated over the years. Finally, there is no substitute for natural lighting and a walk outdoors in the sunshine, even for half an hour a day, for many have antidepressant effects in SAD and perhaps other types of depression as well.

Dark Therapy

Having extolled the benefits of increasing the amount of environmental light, I hesitate to confuse matters by mentioning that for some depressed people, an opposite solution may solve the problem, that is, increasing the daily exposure to darkness.

Dr. Thomas Wehr at the National Institute of Mental Health has suggested that a cause of depression in some people may be our use of artificial lighting to shorten the hours of darkness to which we are exposed each day. Certain people, he argues, may be physically unable to cope with the legacy of Thomas Edison—universal illumination of the night—and may benefit by having the night returned to its natural length. By adopting this strategy in one man, a middle-aged engineer who had cycled in and out of depression for years, Dr. Wehr and colleagues kept him free of depression for many months simply by asking him to remain in darkness for twelve to fourteen hours each day. Since then a few other individuals have derived similar benefit from this treatment. Although at this time, extending the hours of darkness remains an experimental and highly novel treatment that may benefit only a few of those patients who cycle in and out of depression, it is another demonstration of the importance of the environment in regulating mood and the value of manipulating the environment as part of an overall treatment plan for depression.

Strictly Avoid Frightening Ideas

In depressed people the most frightening ideas do not generally come from fear of the outside world but result from turning the darkened lens of depression toward the interior and finding it to be full of self-doubt, self-criticism, guilt, recriminations about the past, and grim predictions for the future. All of these thoughts are not only symptoms of depression but, according to what is called the "cognitive theory of depression" developed by Dr. Aaron Beck and others, can actually propagate the depression and make it worse. Based on this theory, these researchers have developed a psychotherapeutic approach to depression that has actually been shown to be as effective as antidepressant medications in some studies of mild to moderate depression. Cognitive therapy does not advocate avoiding frightening thoughts, but rather adopting a process of reasoning that makes them less so.

Cognitive therapists have developed a way of breaking down depressive thinking into its different components and showing that once you recognize these specific types of depressive thoughts, you can actively work to overcome them. For example, these therapists have accurately recognized the tendency of depressed people to engage in what they refer to as "all or none thinking." With this thinking, a depressed person may regard a project that was not a dazzling success as a total failure. Most ventures in life are not total successes or failures but some mix of the two. A positive attitude enables a person to enjoy those elements of the mix that are successful while learning from the failed elements and then moving on to the next project. This is very hard for the depressed person, who is likely to expend valuable time and energy obsessing about, and magnifying, the failure. The depressed person has difficulty in modulating responses to all sorts of stimuli.

Several other specific distortions of the depressed mind are also worth noting. One is overgeneralization. A depressed person who makes an error is quite likely to think, "You see, nothing I ever do succeeds." Cognitive therapy would seek to challenge this distortion by encouraging the depressed person to find areas in life where he or she has clearly succeeded. Overgeneralization is commonly seen following rejection. A depressed person is likely to take a single rejection as a sign that nobody will ever accept him or her. A healthier approach would be to accept that rejection is part of life and that a single rejection does not necessarily mean that others will follow. Excessive sensitivity to rejection can affect people at any age or stage of life, whether it be the child looking for a friend in the school yard, the adolescent calling someone for a date, or the adult applying for a job or submitting a manuscript or proposal to a publisher or granting agency. Nobody enjoys being rejected, but we can develop ways of putting it into perspective and recognizing that further efforts might well be rewarded with acceptance. After being rejected a depressive person might avoid taking new initiatives for fear of further rejections, thereby greatly diminishing the likelihood of future success. Once again, the depressed person's intellect can be recruited to help understand that this type of thinking is a costly distortion that can be corrected with proper guidance and systematic efforts.

One of the most painful aspects of overgeneralization is that it gets projected into the future. "I will never succeed," "No one will ever love me," or "I will never find happiness" are common distortions of this type that greatly add to feelings of sadness and pessimism. Such distortions have been labeled "fortune-telling" by cognitive therapists, a term that conveys the sense of assurance that a fortune-teller might offer about the future when plain sense indicates that there are too many imponderables to make such predictions with any degree of reliability. This can be pointed out repeatedly by a skillful cognitive therapist, to good effect. Allied to this magical depressive tendency to fortune-telling is "mind reading," a process by which the depressed person thinks and talks as though he or she can read what is in another person's mind. So a depressed person might say, "She didn't want to come on a date with me because she thinks I am too dull and nerdy," or an unsuccessful applicant may say, "He didn't accept me for the job because I'm not qualified." The cognitive therapist will point out that other possible explanations for these outcomes abound. The girl who declined to go out on a date with you may already be committed to someone else; the prospective employer may have an inside candidate in mind for the job, and so on. Bearing in mind these alternative possible explanations empowers the rejected person, who is then more easily able to pursue other possibilities. In contrast, depressive thinking tends to paralyze the thinker, increasing his or her sense of powerlessness and reducing enthusiasm for making further efforts, which might be more successful.

In summary, it is important to recognize and address frightening thoughts, more technically known as "depressive distortions." Fortunately, treatment strategies have been developed to tackle such thoughts and these strategies work if they are implemented diligently and systematically. For those interested in learning more about cognitive therapy, I recommend the book *Feeling Good* by David Burns (see "Selected Bibliography and Further Reading").

Cultivate All Types of Healthy Pleasures

Many of the suggestions of A. Cornelius Celsus mentioned earlier in this chapter are healthy pleasures—music, soothing sounds like that of running water, cheerful conversations, massage, and travel. Whatever it is that is a source of pleasure should be sought out and developed by the depressed person because the essence of depression is the lack of capacity for enjoyment, also known as anhedonia. But even when a certain degree of anhedonia is present, some activities might still provide pleasure.

Pets, for example, can be a great source of comfort and delight even to depressed people. Many years ago I decided that it would be a useful exercise to put several of my depressed patients together in a group. I reasoned that they might be able to help one another cope with depression. In truth, it was not a good idea. The group was suffused by a sense of communal gloom and despair. But I remember on one occasion, when someone mentioned her dog or cat, there was an immediate change in atmosphere as each of the group members pulled out a picture of his or her pet—animals that until that moment I had in some instances not even known existed. For some time they pored over one another's pictures, admiring the animals and discussing their various special qualities and foibles. It was a vivid demonstration to me of the power of animals to cheer people up, and how even depressed people are capable of spells of happiness if they are presented with the right stimuli.

Only you know what it is that delights you most when you are feeling well and how best to seek out such activities. Ask yourself what it is that still appeals even though you may be depressed. Is it painting watercolors, growing orchids, or taking long walks in the countryside? The possibilities are limited only by the imagination. Consider the question, make a list of such sources of joy, and then devise strategies for how you can bring healthy pleasures back into your life again.

I specify healthy pleasures because some pleasures are quite unhealthy, even if they are capable of bringing you out of depression for brief periods. Such pleasures include alcohol and addictive drugs and compulsive behaviors, such as excessive shopping, spending, gambling, or illicit sexual activity. One of my depressed patients, for example, would regularly shop for clothes that she could ill afford, did not need, and, in fact, hardly ever wore. Her closet was full of expensive dresses that she had never even tried on after leaving the store. For her, all the reward came from the act of shopping itself. There was something about the process of going to an expensive store, trying on the garment, and having the saleslady pay attention to her and compliment her that proved irresistible. Of course, the comfort was very short-lived and the cost of the habit, both financially and in the form of marital conflict, severely exacerbated her depression. There are many different varieties of this habit and they can be very difficult to break. Addictive sexual behavior is another costly way in which some people medicate their depressed feelings. At times I have recommended specific recovery groups for these types of problems with fairly good results.

And how do you tell the difference between a healthy pleasure and an unhealthy one? Usually it is fairly obvious. The one leaves you feeling good afterward; the other leaves you feeling bad. The one feels like a wise investment that continues to yield dividends over time; the other like a foolish expenditure of time, money, and energy, which ends up costing more than it's worth. And, finally, the one is a source of pride that you might be pleased to share with friends and family, whereas the other is often a source of shame, cloaked in secrecy.

Get Help

One of my favorite *New Yorker* cartoons consists of two panels. In the first panel a drowning woman cries out to her sheepdog at the edge of the lake, "Get help, Lassie, get help." The next panel shows the obedient dog lying on an analyst's couch.

Getting help does not always mean subjecting yourself to deep psychological examination. It can be quite concrete. An overwhelmed mother might find it invaluable to get more help with baby-sitting or housework. An overwhelmed student might need some special tutoring. Depressed people—like all who are ill—often feel overwhelmed by what they have to do but are ashamed or reluctant to reach out and ask for help. If you had a backache or hepatitis, you wouldn't think twice about getting help so that your life might become more manageable. Well, depression is just as legitimate a condition, even if there are no X rays or lab tests to validate it. Part of getting better is accepting that you are suffering from a medical illness—depression. As one patient put it, "Just understanding what is going on is half the battle." Once you accept that fact, you will feel better about taking all the steps needed to help you feel better again, including reaching out to those who can make life easier for you.

12

FREQUENTLY ASKED QUESTIONS ABOUT ST. JOHN'S WORT AND A PRACTICAL GUIDE TO ITS USE

In materia medica, the deductions of clinical experience often precede those of scientific analysis, and science sometimes comes later to inform us why we produce certain effects with medicines. Practice, based on clear scientific deductions, is, of course, the most desirable; but this we cannot always wait for. If a remedy long outlives what may be termed its fashionable existence and still maintains a reputation for definite remedial effects, it is reasonable to infer that such properties are not imaginary.

—F. A. BURRELL, "SOME USES OF THE OLEUM HYPERICI," *NEW ENGLAND MEDICAL MONTHLY*, 1887

These words, written over a hundred years ago about the use of an extract of St. John's wort, are as relevant today as they were then. Although numerous scientific studies on the clinical and pharmacological effects of the herb have been published, there are many questions that have a direct bearing on clinical practice for which we do not at this time have definitive scientific answers. In the meantime, however, until these questions are answered at the level of definitive science, those who are interested in using the herb want to get the best information available to answer certain questions they may have about it.

Fortunately, we have a wealth of clinical and anecdotal experience with St. John's wort, which has been used as an herbal remedy for centuries. In the past decade, millions of prescriptions for St. John's wort have been written in Germany, and large numbers of people have purchased the herb over the counter and have taken it of their own accord. The growing popularity of St. John's wort in the United States has allowed clinicians and researchers such as myself to evaluate some of the questions that are on the minds of people considering the remedy for themselves and to come up with working solutions that have immediate practical implications. In this chapter, I address some of the most commonly asked questions about St. John's wort and its use.

In answering some of the most frequently asked questions about St. John's wort, I have drawn not only on the literature and my own clinical experience with the herb but also on reports obtained through an informal survey and from interviews with some of the leading experts in Europe on the herbal antidepressant. I have been assisted specifically by Drs. Siegfried Kasper, Hans-Peter Volz, and Franz Müller-Spahn, chiefs of the departments of psychiatry in Vienna, Austria; Jena, Germany; and Basel, Switzerland; and Dr. David Wheatley, who has conducted clinical trials of the herbal antidepressant in England.

What Is St. John's Wort?

For a description of St. John's wort, the plant, also known as *Hypericum perforatum*, I can do no better than to quote Dr. O. Phelps Brown who wrote in 1885:

This is a beautiful shrub, and is a great adornment to our meadows. It has a hard and woody root, which abides in the ground many years, shooting anew every year. The stalks run up about two feet high, spreading many branches, having deep-green, ovate, obtuse and opposite leaves, which are full of small holes, which are plainly seen when the leaf is held up to the light. At the tops of the stalks and branches stand yellow flowers of five leaves apiece with many yellow threads in the middle, which, being bruised, yield a reddish juice, like blood, after which come small round heads, wherein is contained small blackish seed, smelling like resin.

This description comes from a book titled *The Complete Herbalist; or The People, Their Own Physicians by the Use of Nature's Remedies; Describing the Great Curative Properties Found in the Herbal Kingdom*. Over a hundred years ago, it seems, people were intrigued by the same possibilities that we are revisiting today—of using nature's apothecary as a source of remedies and of healing oneself instead of always seeking out the assistance of a physician.

The pores in the leaves of St. John's wort, which look like perforations and give the plant half of its botanical name (*perforatum*), are thought to contain the plant's pharmacologically active substances, as are the black spots on the petals. It is these black spots which, when rubbed, yield a reddish liquid that was used for dying clothes in earlier times.

How Are the Active Ingredients Obtained from the Plant?

The active ingredients have been extracted from the plant in various ways over the ages. One folk remedy, used even in modern times, is to brew a tea out of the leaves and flowers. The seventeenth-century chemist Angelo Sala originally used brandy to extract the active essence. In modern times, commercial companies still use a form of alcohol to extract the active ingredients, which they then enclose in a pill or capsule.

Which Are the Active Antidepressant Substances in St. John's Wort?

At this time, no one knows the answer to this question for sure. In the course of evolution, the plant appears to have developed the capacity to produce many compounds that have pharmacological effects in humans and animals. Some of these substances are toxic to animals and in this way might have served to protect the plant over millennia of evolution. We know, for example, that cattle that eat too much of the plant can develop harmful or even fatal skin reactions when they are subsequently exposed to sunlight. I should emphasize that these harmful doses are dozens of times greater than the doses used for treating depression, which are quite safe.

Most of the research on St. John's wort, both with depressed patients and in the laboratory, has been performed with an extract of St. John's wort called LI 160. This extract contains many active substances. Although most attention has been focused on two of these substances—hypericin and pseudohypericin—more attention is now being paid to a third substance, hyperforin, which appears to have some of the pharmacological properties thought to be responsible for the effects of the herb as a whole. In an herb containing such a complex mixture of active compounds, it is quite possible that more than one of the compounds is having a therapeutic effect and that they are acting in harmony to complement one another's actions.

Does the Brand of St. John's Wort That You Use Make a Difference?

The simple answer to this question is yes.

Professor Hanns Hippius, formerly director of the psychiatric clinic at Ludwig-Maximilian University in Munich, Germany, writes:

The 1996 German list of available drugs, the *Rote Liste*, includes 28 Hypericum preparations. Since these preparations are not chemically defined single-substances or combination preparations, but whole extracts of the St. John's wort plant, it cannot automatically be assumed that the various medicinal preparations from various

manufacturers have the same composition and therefore the same therapeutic efficacy at the same dosage.

I agree with Dr. Hippius. In other words, since we do not
know which substances in St. John's wort are responsible for
its antidepressant effects, we cannot assume that all plant
preparations are equivalent, even if the amount of hypericin,
which is supposedly standardized across different preparations, is the same. I say "supposedly" based on my experience
with the use of certain generic antidepressants. Generic antidepressants are supposed to have the same amount and quality of
the active compound as the original brand-name products. Yet
I have often observed a relapse of depressive symptoms in
patients who have previously been doing very well when they
switch from a certain brand-name antidepressant to its generic
counterpart. If different brands of a synthetic compound produced under the supervision of the Food and Drug
Administration result in different clinical effects, how much
more reason do we have to doubt the equivalency of different
herbal products with their complex combinations of active substances and produced under much looser regulatory conditions? Consider, for example, how wines that are made from
the same type of grape will vary in taste not only from one
country or region to another but even from vintage to vintage.
The substances in the wine that imbue it with its special bou-
quet and flavor will change with the soil, the amount of sunshine, and the rainfall. A similar situation can be expected to
apply to the composition of an extract of St. John's wort, where
the variable of interest is not the flavor but rather the antidepressant effects or the side effects of the preparation.

Once we acknowledge that herbal preparations are likely to
vary in their composition, where does that leave us in terms of
choosing the best preparation? At this point there have been no
actual studies comparing one type of St. John's wort preparation to another. Yet most of the research in which the antidepressant effects of St. John's wort have been established has
been performed using the Jarsin brand, produced by Lichtwer

Pharma, the leading German manufacturer of the herbal remedy. This has led clinician and researcher Hans-Peter Volz to conclude that "taken in sum, the antidepressive action of hypericum is only sufficiently documented for Jarsin."

The good news is that Jarsin is now available over the counter in the United States under the brand name Kira. It is essentially identical to the German compound and is clearly the brand of choice at this time.

Another reason to use an herbal product known to be made under carefully supervised conditions is that you can feel more confident that there are no potentially toxic contaminants, such as have been known to appear in certain other food supplements. The contaminant in a certain formulation of L-tryptophan that resulted in several fatalities was a particularly dramatic case in point.

Some other brands of St. John's wort are less expensive than Kira and for certain individuals the cost difference may be a significant consideration. If this is the case, I would suggest at least starting with the Kira brand. If your depression does not respond, you can then be more confident that it is not because of the brand of the herbal remedy but for other reasons. Once your depression does respond to Kira, if cost is a significant consideration, you might then try to switch to a less expensive brand and see if you maintain the same level of antidepressant response.

What Types of Depressions Respond Best to St. John's Wort?

St. John's wort should be considered as a first-line treatment for:
- mild depression
- short-term stress associated with depression and anxiety
- moderate depression
- depression in those who are very sensitive to, or concerned about, side effects

- winter depression (seasonal affective disorder, or **SAD**)
- depression in the elderly
- dysthymia (chronic low-grade unhappiness)

St. John's wort should be considered, but probably not as a first-line treatment, for:

- depression in children and adolescents
- severe depression

St. John's wort should not be considered for:

- depression in pregnancy

As I discussed in chapter 4, the beneficial effects of the herb have been most convincingly demonstrated for mild and moderate depressions. In the 1997 study by Dr. Vorbach and colleagues, it was used in more severely depressed individuals and proved roughly as effective as the standard antidepressant imipramine. More research will be needed, however, before the herbal remedy can be recommended for more severe depressions.

A severely depressed man consulted me recently. He had legal actions pending against him and was in danger of being put in jail. His business was in disarray and he was struggling to manage his day-to-day affairs. His desk was covered in papers and he was unable to muster the will or concentration to deal with them. He could hardly sleep at all and it was an effort to fight his way through his exhaustion and get through each day. Yet it was critical that he be as functional as possible in order to cooperate with his lawyer in reaching the best possible deal with his creditors and the prosecutor's office. He also needed to be alert and active in keeping his business afloat and avoiding bankruptcy if at all possible. He needed my help urgently. Given the seriousness of my patient's depression, he was not someone on whom I wanted to try something that had not been fully researched for severe depression. I therefore chose a more established antidepressant, nortriptyline, to which my patient responded well within a few weeks. Nortriptyline is one of a family of potent older antidepressants, which may have a number of undesirable side effects such as dry mouth, constipation, and blurred vision. These side effects seemed like reasonable trade-offs given the seriousness of this patient's predicament. If the situation had been less urgent, however, I would have been more inclined to administer the herbal antidepressant because of its much lower likelihood of producing unpleasant side effects.

As more research studies are performed on the use of St. John's wort for serious depression, clinical reasoning might change and the herbal antidepressant might emerge as a first-line treatment even for severe depressions. In my experience, severely depressed people often end up on more than one anti-depressant, and there is no reason why St. John's wort should not be used as one of a combination of antidepressants if more than one is required. The use of St. John's wort in the treatment of SAD and depression in the elderly has been discussed in detail elsewhere (see chapters 6 and 7).

It is only relatively recently that clinicians and the public at large have become aware of how common depression is in children and adolescents. There has been a rapid increase in the prescription of antidepressants for young patients in recent years. Because there have not as yet been any studies on the use of St. John's wort in young people, the herbal remedy should not be considered as a first-line treatment for these individuals. Nevertheless, I know of some cases where the herb has been used effectively in adolescents and have described one such case in an earlier chapter. In depressed children and adolescents, St. John's wort should be regarded as a second-line treatment, to be used if conventional antidepressants prove unsuitable for any reason.

Treating pregnant women with medications is something always undertaken with hesitancy and only after very careful deliberation given the possibility that any medication may affect the growth and development of the baby. Yet some pregnant women are so depressed that it seems wrong not to provide them with relief for their symptoms because of some theoretical risk to the baby. In such cases I try to use medications with the longest track record, particularly if there is published literature on their safe use in pregnancy. No such literature exists for the use of St. John's wort in pregnant women, whereas there is some reassuring evidence that the older antidepressants, and Prozac, might be relatively safe for the developing baby. I would therefore prefer to use these drugs rather than St. John's wort for the treatment of depression in pregnancy.

How Much St. John's Wort Should I Use? How Many Times Per Day Do I Need to Take It?

Most studies of the antidepressant effects of St. John's wort have used one 300-mg tablet three times per day. In my experience with using many other antidepressants, however, I have been impressed by the wide variation in dosage required by different people. To some degree, this relates to the ability of a person's liver to break down the antidepressant into inactive substances, which are then excreted. This ability varies tremendously from person to person. To some extent, one can get an indication of how sensitive a person is going to be to a new medication by reviewing that person's sensitivity to medications in the past. The amount of medication needed is often not related to the size of the person being treated. I have been impressed over the years by small female patients who have been able to tolerate enormous dosages of antidepressants, in contrast to very large men who have been sensitive to tiny dosages.

I believe that there will be a range of optimal dosages for St. John's wort as well. A good practical way to begin treatment is to:

- Start with one tablet a day, with breakfast, for two to three days.

- Follow up by taking two tablets a day (one with breakfast and one with lunch) for a further two to three days.

- Then take three tablets a day (one each with breakfast, lunch, and dinner).

- Stay on that dosage for several weeks unless side effects require a reduction in dosage.

The reason I like to begin with a low dosage is that whereas therapeutic effects often take weeks to appear, the side effects of any antidepressant may occur very soon after first taking it. If this should happen, one is always better off having taken a small rather than a large dosage. In addition, it sometimes takes awhile for your system to get used to a new medication, and gradually increasing the dosage gives your system a chance to adjust to it. I should mention, however, that it is standard practice in Germany to begin with one St. John's wort tablet three times a day.

- Taking medications with meals reduces the likelihood of developing gastrointestinal side effects such as nausea, indigestion, or abdominal pains, which may occur with St. John's wort. The meal will not interfere with the effects of the treatment in any way.

- If you should develop side effects after increasing the dosage to, say, two pills a day but the side effects are mild, try to remain on that dosage for at least a few days. Side effects may settle down within a few days. If you increase the dosage without waiting for this to happen, the side effects may get worse and this may discourage you from staying on the medication. It may turn out that the current dosage will be just right for you. Alternatively, if this dosage proves to be too low, once the side effects diminish sufficiently you may be able to increase the dosage at a later time if you need to.

- You may be able to get by with taking St. John's wort less frequently than three times a day. Taking a medication three times a day can be quite inconvenient. Somehow the midday dosage often gets skipped. It is generally much easier to take medications twice a day and some people have found that a twice-daily dosage of St. John's wort (two pills at breakfast and one at dinner) works well for them. One or two of my patients developed indigestion when they used the herb in this way and found that taking it three times a day with meals completely resolved that side effect. If you should happen to forget the midday dosage, however, it is preferable to double the evening dose rather than skip one dose for the day, bringing the day's total to three St. John's wort tablets. Because no one is sure of what the active ingredients are in St. John's wort, it is impossible at this time to say what the best dosing schedule really is and more research is required to answer this question. At this time, I recommend that you start using St. John's wort three times a day and, later on, after you have established that it works for you, it may be worth experimenting with different dosing schedules. It is possible that for some people, like the man whose wife mixed his St. John's wort with his breakfast vitamins, a once-a-day schedule will prove to be sufficient.

- You may need more than three tablets of St. John's wort (900 mg) per day. Just as it is possible that some people will not need three St. John's wort tablets per day but may respond fully to one or two tablets, so others may require more than three tablets per day.

- It is probably worth staying on three tablets per day for at least five weeks before deciding to increase the dosage.

- In one study of more serious depression, 1,800 mg of hypericum (six tablets) proved to be roughly as effective as a conventional antidepressant, and the researcher running the study remarked that the frequency of side effects did not appear to be greater than he had encountered on the more conventional lower dosage of three tablets per day.

It would be surprising to me if, just as with other antidepressants, different people did not end up needing different amounts of hypericum and I would encourage you and your doctor to experiment with different dosages up to 1,800 mg (six tablets per day) provided you do not experience any particularly unpleasant side effects and provided you give the lower dosage of 900 mg (three tablets) a fair trial of five to six weeks before increasing the dosage.

How Long After Starting St. John's Wort Should I Expect to See an Improvement?

Although some people may experience relief from the symptoms of depression within days of starting St. John's wort, for others it may be as long as six weeks before there is a real sense of improvement. An informal survey of European psychiatrists who have treated hundreds of patients with St. John's wort revealed that most believe that one should wait at least three weeks after a full dose (900 mg per day) of St. John's wort has been started before judging whether it has been effective or not. In this regard, St. John's wort is similar to other antidepressants, most of which take between two and four weeks to produce their initial antidepressant effects. The reason for this delay in response to antidepressants has been the focus of considerable research, but at this time no one has really come up with a satisfactory explanation for it. If you detect no benefit after three weeks, you have the choice of increasing the dosage of St. John's wort, switching to a conventional antidepressant, or adding the antidepressant to the St. John's wort dosage.

How Can I Monitor My Response to St. John's Wort?

Depression is by its very nature a discouraging condition, and the response to antidepressants in general is often not smooth and linear. Your mood can bob up and down, and it may be hard to tell just where you are compared to where you were before you started treatment. In my practice I have used a very simple method to help my patients monitor their moods over time. On pages 217–218 is a simple form that will help you to chart your mood in response to starting St. John's wort. Just as when you diet, it is helpful to weigh yourself regularly so as to see the pattern of response, so it can be very helpful to chart your mood on a weekly basis after you start a new type of antidepressant treatment. And just as when you diet, you can gain a pound or two on a particular day, perhaps as a result of water retention, even though you are succeeding in losing weight over the long run, so it is possible to have one or two bad days even though your mood may be better overall. Being able to refer to the chart is helpful in illustrating this overall improvement. Alternatively, if you are not improving, you might be inclined to try and kid yourself into thinking that you are. Referring to the chart may reveal that not to be so and prompt you to shift your strategy to find a different way out of your depression.

Watch Out for a Partial Response

Let's say that you have been taking St. John's wort for several weeks and that there is no question that you are feeling better. Perhaps you can even see the difference on your mood chart. Should you be satisfied and ask no further questions? Not necessarily. This might be the time to get greedy. When I treat patients in my own practice, I am very ambitious for them, by which I mean that I want them to feel as well as they possibly can and I try to convey that sense of ambition to them. If they are feeling quite good, perhaps they could do even better. The reason for this approach is that it is often difficult to know when a depression has been fully treated. Often there is such relief that the intense pain of depression—the dark, heavy, dismal, dreary sense of pessimism and despair—has lifted that what remains seems just fine by comparison. Yet there may still be a sense of fatigue, low energy, and insufficient optimism, drive, or zest for life that may signal that elements of the depression remain. It is important to look for such elements because there is a good chance that further treatment, such as increasing dosage or adding another medication, might remove all vestiges of the depression. A psychiatrist friend of mine is fond of saying that you never know when you have enough until you have too much. Although he is referring to life in general, the same is often true about treating depression as fully as possible. Of course, if side effects are already present, it might not pay to increase dosage or add medications. That is where a careful cost-benefit analysis is in order to weigh the potential value of further antidepressant effects against the potential liability of more side effects.

In addition to using chemical or herbal antidepressants, don't forget the array of lifestyle changes that you can make that will greatly enhance the effects of any of these medications, including St. John's wort, as I have discussed in the previous chapter.

What If I Am Feeling Suicidal?

Suicidal feelings are not a suitable condition for self-help remedies—no ifs, ands, or buts. If you are feeling suicidal, you definitely need to reach out for the help of others and should certainly consult a qualified professional. That does not mean that you cannot take and benefit from St. John's wort. It does mean that it's too risky for you to do so on your own without the careful and caring guidance of others. It has been said that suicide is a permanent solution to a temporary problem. Better solutions can always be found and I urge you to consult a good doctor who can help you to find them.

Can St. John's Wort Be Used in the Treatment of Bipolar Depression, Also Known As Manic Depression?

People with recurrent depressions can be divided into unipolar and bipolar categories. Those with recurrent unipolar depressions suffer only from periods of low mood, separated from one another by normal periods. In contrast, those with bipolar depression experience periods of exaggerated energy and activity as well as depressions. During their activated periods, known as manic or hypomanic (less severe than manic) episodes, these individuals need less sleep, think and talk more quickly, and are more sped up than normal. Sometimes they are elated, but at other times are quite irritable and angry, especially when they feel blocked, frustrated, or thwarted by those around them, who appear to them to be moving at a snail's pace. The question here is whether a bipolar person can safely use St. John's wort during a period of depression.

Unfortunately, there are as yet no published studies on the use of St. John's wort in the treatment of bipolar depression. We do, however, know two important facts about the treatment of bipolar depression with other antidepressants: (1) All antidepressants that work in the treatment of unipolar depression also work for bipolar depression; and (2) all antidepressants are capable of inducing hypomanic or manic episodes in patients with bipolar depression. Based on these observations, I would expect St. John's wort to be an effective antidepressant in bipolar depressions. I would also caution anyone with a tendency to develop hypomanic or manic symptoms to be sure to use the herbal antidepressant only under the close supervision of a physician and on no account to experiment with its use on your own. In addition, in most bipolar patients, it is customary to use a mood stabilizer such as lithium carbonate or valproic acid before adding an antidepressant to guard against the development of a hypomanic or manic episode. For those of you who are wondering why one should be so careful to prevent the development of a hypomanic or manic episode, I should mention that they can be extremely disruptive and destructive to a person's life. Even though a mild hypomanic episode may not be harmful, when the process reaches its extremes, it can cause the breakup of a marriage, the loss of a job, serious financial reversals, and physical injury to the affected person.

To my knowledge, there have been no published reports of manic episodes induced by St. John's wort, and there is no greater reason to be concerned about the herbal remedy in this regard than about any other effective antidepressant. Even so, it is good to be aware of the potential risk, especially if you have a history of hypomania or mania. One of my patients who has experienced recurrent depressions and mild hypomanias in the past is on a maintenance dose of lithium carbonate to stabilize his moods. When he developed a mild depression, I started him on two tablets of St. John's wort per day. A week later he called me to say that he was feeling "too good" and waking up in the early hours of the morning. I interpreted this as possible evidence of hypomania and suggested that he cut back to one tablet a day, which turned out to be just the right amount for him. Another case of possible hypomania induced by St. John's wort was brought to my attention by a colleague. Once you are aware of the possibility that hypomania can develop with the use of any antidepressant, you are forewarned and better able to deal with the symptoms should they arise.

What Side Effects Might I Expect in Using St. John's Wort?

The best data base on side effects comes from a large German study in which over 3,000 patients on St. John's wort were monitored by their physicians, over 650 of whom participated in the survey. Only 48 patients (about 1.5 percent) discontinued the medication in the study, and side effects were reported by only 79 people (2.4 percent). Of these side effects, the most commonly reported problems were gastrointestinal irritation, restlessness, and allergic reactions, all of which were reported by less than 1 percent. European experts whom I have interviewed about St. John's wort's side effects agree with these very low percentages. Such low side-effect frequencies are especially good news for the treatment of depression in the elderly, who are typically highly susceptible to the side effects of all sorts of medications.

Although time will tell whether the initial observations of such low frequencies of side effects are correct, I have been impressed in my own clinical practice by the absence of any side effects in some people who have proved to be highly sensitive to side effects from a wide variety of other antidepressants. It seems likely that St. John's wort will indeed prove to have fewer side effects than the synthetic antidepressants currently in use.

As noted above, anyone with a history of hypomanic or manic episodes should be especially vigilant to the typical symptoms of activation after starting any antidepressant. Sleeplessness, racing thoughts, pressured speech, and euphoria or irritability are early warning signs of hypomania or mania that must be heeded. If these develop, you should stop St. John's wort immediately and consult a physician. The loss of sleep (which is often not experienced as unpleasant but rather as an extra opportunity to get more accomplished or have more fun) is harmful in itself, as it can fuel the manic process. If caught early, the symptoms of hypomania or mania can often be checked with appropriate actions; if not, however, they can escalate into mania, which can be very unpleasant and damaging.

A few of my patients have developed increased anxiety after beginning St. John's wort. Such reactions have also been reported to occur in certain individuals after starting other types of antidepressants. People with a history of panic attacks or extreme anxiety are especially susceptible in this regard. Yet antidepressants have actually been given for the treatment of anxiety and panic. In order to overcome the initial anxiety response, which may occur after taking even a single dose, it is necessary to back down on the dosage. For example, in treating such sensitive patients with Prozac, I have often started with as little as 1 to 2 mg of liquid Prozac per day—one tenth of the standard dose. After the person has become used to that dosage, it is then possible to increase the dosage slowly and carefully over the ensuing weeks until a therapeutic level is reached. If you are eager to persevere with St. John's wort but happen to develop anxiety after taking a tablet or two, it is possible to overcome the problem by obtaining an herbal extract in the form of a liquid, known as an elixir. Two reputable companies that distribute an elixir of St. John's wort are Herb Pharm and Gaia. Begin by taking very low dosages of the elixir (say, one tenth of the recommended number of drops) and increase gradually at a rate that you can comfortably tolerate until you reach therapeutic levels.

Some people on St. John's wort have complained about increased sensitivity to sunlight both with regard to the skin, with more reddening occurring than usual, and the eyes. At this time there is no reason to believe that either of these side effects is of clinical concern, but if they cause discomfort, protection of the skin with sunblock or the eyes with sunglasses would be a sensible preventive measure.

Should I Switch from the Antidepressant I Am Taking to St. John's Wort?

The answer to this question depends on how you are doing on your present medication. If the medication is working with few or no side effects, why switch? You are lucky to have found something that works well for you. As the old maxim goes, if it ain't broke, don't fix it. On the other hand, if the medication is not working well or is causing bothersome side effects, you have good reason to be considering a switch to St. John's wort.

How Do I Switch from Another Antidepressant to St. John's Wort?

If you are already on another antidepressant and are considering switching to St. John's wort, there are certain considerations worth bearing in mind. First, the other antidepressant has presumably been prescribed by a physician and it is wise to inform that physician about what you would like to do. This should not be construed as asking the physician's permission. As an adult, it is hardly necessary for you to do so. It is nevertheless not only a courtesy, but also of practical value as you might need to return to that physician for advice or help of one sort or another if your experiment does not work out. In that case, it will be much easier to elicit the physician's help if it does not appear as though you have been off on a frolic of your own. In addition, if the physician is competent and knowledgeable, he or she might provide you with invaluable advice that will supplement the advice provided here and customize it to your particular needs. If the physician is not open-minded about new treatments, you may wish to consider seeing another doctor.

Second, as I have already noted, it is almost always useful when switching from one medication to another to do so gradually, tapering the one while starting the other, thus overlapping the two medications, which can be used in conjunction in the transition period. Exceptions to this rule are when the medication you are on is causing serious side effects, in which case you might need to stop it abruptly, or if the two medications are not compatible with each other (about which, more below). Even though antidepressants as a group are not addictive and people do not generally experience severe withdrawal on stopping them, abruptly discontinuing them may result in unpleasant symptoms such as interrupted sleep or flulike feelings. For some people these are worse than for others. For example, a few of my patients have developed the feeling that they are having electric shocks to their body after discontinuing the antidepressant Paxil. One factor worth bearing in mind in discontinuing a medication is its half-life. The half-life of a medication is the time required, after a single dose is taken, for the level of that medication in the bloodstream to drop from the maximum level to half that level. A drug like Prozac, for example, with a long half-life, persists in the system for many days after the drug is discontinued and is less likely to cause symptoms on withdrawal. The drug Effexor, on the other hand, has a very short half-life, is excreted from the system in a matter of hours rather than days, and is more likely to result in symptoms following withdrawal. In general, withdrawal symptoms are more marked when one discontinues a drug with a shorter as opposed to a longer half-life. In addition to withdrawal symptoms, you risk experiencing a nasty relapse of your depressive symptoms after discontinuing an antidepressant. In any event, it is generally best to discontinue antidepressant medication gradually rather than abruptly.

Two antidepressants may influence each other in ways that are sometimes predictable but often are not. For example, they may enhance each other's beneficial or adverse effects. For this reason, it is often best if they are not coadministered in their full dosage strength.

Say, for example, that you are on Zoloft, 100 mg per day, and want to switch to St. John's wort, 900 mg (three tablets) per day. It might make sense to drop to 50 mg per day of Zoloft while adding one tablet of St. John's wort per day for a period of three to four days. After that interval, if there are no ill effects, you might add a second tablet of St. John's wort together with the 50 mg of Zoloft for a further four days. At the end of the second week, depending on how you are feeling, it might be reasonable to shift to the full 900 mg of St. John's wort (three tablets) and stop the Zoloft altogether. You might expect some mood instability or side effects during this transition time because levels of Zoloft will be dropping in your blood as levels of St. John's wort are increasing, but these symptoms should be easily manageable. If they are not, slow down the process. As you can see, it is really best to have a good physician to guide, accompany, and befriend you through this transition process. With Prozac you might want to double the intervals noted above because Prozac has a much longer half-life than Zoloft, which means it lingers in the system for longer periods of time.

Other medications might need to be handled somewhat differently depending on the half-lives of the medications and their particular properties.

Note: If you are on a monoamine oxidase inhibitor (MAOI) such as Nardil or Parnate, the type of medication that prohibits eating yellow cheese or drinking red wine, the above rules of transition do not apply. You need to wait a full two weeks after completely discontinuing the MAOI before starting treatment with St. John's wort.

Can I Combine St. John's Wort with Other Antidepressant Medications?

As I have already mentioned, it is possible to administer St. John's wort with a variety of other antidepressants and other medications in general. A survey of European colleagues who have treated collectively several hundred patients with St. John's wort revealed no drug interactions noted to date except for potential problematic interactions with the MAOIs, as noted above. At one point it was thought that St. John's wort might itself be an MAOI and might exert its antidepressant effects by that mechanism. If that were the case, it would be potentially dangerous to combine St. John's wort with other antidepressants. Fortunately, that does not appear to be the case to any significant degree, and St. John's wort can be used in combination with antidepressants other than the MAOIs, provided this is done carefully and under a doctor's supervision. Furthermore, based on the best information available to date, you need not worry if you are taking St. John's wort that you will develop the extremely uncomfortable and sometimes dangerous high blood pressure reaction after eating cheese or drinking red wine, as can occur with those who are on an MAOI.

You might be best off moving more gradually with dosages if St. John's wort is used in combination with other antidepressants or stimulants, as these medications all act on the nerve cells in the brain and can enhance one another's effects. While this is one of the desired goals of the exercise, namely, to induce a more powerful antidepressant effect than would be obtained on any of the medications alone, it is also a reason to increase dosages gradually to avoid the development of exaggerated and unduly unpleasant side effects.

What Is the "Serotonin Syndrome," and Can It Occur on St. John's Wort?

The serotonin syndrome is a cluster of symptoms that occurs when there is too much serotonin in brain synapses. Although it has occurred most commonly when the MAOIs are combined with other drugs or substances that tend to increase the amount of serotonin in the brain, it can also occur with combinations of medications not involving MAOIs. For example, the serotonin syndrome has been observed at times when the dietary supplement L-tryptophan, the amino acid from which serotonin is synthesized in the brain, is added to a selective serotonin-reuptake inhibitor such as Prozac or when various antidepressants are combined. Because St. John's wort appears to increase the amount of serotonin in the synapse, there are theoretical reasons to believe that it might also cause the serotonin syndrome if combined with other antidepressants.

In fact, a few cases of the serotonin syndrome following combinations of St. John's wort and an antidepressant have now been reported in a psychiatric newsletter. As the herbal remedy is more widely used in combination with other antidepressants, we may see more such cases, but they are likely to be rare. None of the European experts surveyed for this book had encountered the problem, despite using such medication combinations. However, although concerns about the serotonin syndrome need not deter you from combining St. John's wort with other antidepressants under the supervision of a doctor, it is good to be aware of the syndrome's symptoms so that you can report them to your doctor promptly if they occur.

The most common features of the serotonin syndrome are

- confusion
- hypomanic symptoms (such as overactivity, flight of ideas, and pressured speech)
- restlessness
- muscle twitches
- sweating
- shivering
- diarrhea
- poor coordination

If promptly diagnosed and treated, the serotonin syndrome should resolve without any long-term ill effects. If the symptoms are allowed to progress, this complication can be dangerous. To date, no long-term serious consequences have been reported as a result of combining St. John's wort with other antidepressants.

What About Combining St. John's Wort with Alcohol?

Alcohol itself often complicates the treatment of depression. Although depressed people often report a pleasant buzz after using alcohol, in my experience they often pay for this buzz heavily in the days that follow. This delayed effect is often difficult to discern. If your mood is bad to start with and it feels worse on certain days, there are any number of good reasons to explain the mood worsening. The two or three drinks you had last night or the night before are by now a distant memory and hardly seem to be likely culprits. But careful observation in many patients has shown that once the alcohol is stopped, mood control is often much smoother and better. Now, if you enjoy having several drinks of an evening, I hardly expect these mild observations of mine to persuade you to stop doing so, but it's worth thinking about. If you're keeping a mood log, you might note when you drink (including the number and type) and see whether you can detect an impact of the drinks on your mood over the ensuing days.

Quite aside from the potential problem of drinking alcohol if you happen to suffer from depression is the question of whether you can safely drink alcohol if you are on St. John's wort. The answer is that there is no known negative interaction between St. John's wort and alcohol. Even so, I always suggest that my patients go easy on the alcohol if they are on any antidepressant (no more than one or two beers or glasses of wine or one mixed drink is what I usually recommend). After all, if these drugs are all working on the brain, it would be strange if they did not affect each other's actions in one way or another.

How Long Should I Stay on St. John's Wort?

This question could just as easily be asked in relation to any other antidepressant. In one form or another, it is one of the more common questions on the mind of anyone who has felt the benefit of an antidepressant medication. The experience of relief and gratitude is counterbalanced in many people by a sense of unease at having to be on a medication for an undefined and possibly indefinite period of time. The honest answer is that we just can't predict how long someone will need to be on an antidepressant. If the depression has been a single, short-lived episode, it may be possible to stop the antidepressant after six months of remission without risking relapse. If there is a history of repeated episodes or long-standing depression, however, there is a high likelihood that depression will recur or relapse if the antidepressant is stopped. In such people, it generally makes good sense to stay on an antidepressant indefinitely. Although there have been no long-term studies of St. John's wort in depression—and I should say that such studies are few and far between for other antidepressants as well—there is no evidence of any long-term problems in those who have been on St. John's wort for months or even years.

After several months of treatment, people often experiment and stop their antidepressants just to make sure that they still really need them. If you do that, be sure to watch out for early signs of relapse and return to St. John's wort as soon as these appear. It is much easier to reverse the symptoms of depression in their initial stages than after they are fully established again.

Should Everyone Try St. John's Wort?

Our experience with other antidepressants suggests that the answer to this question is no. Although antidepressants, as their name implies, improve mood in people who are suffering from depression, there is no evidence that they are universal "pick-me-ups." Since St. John's wort appears to work in ways that are similar to those of other antidepressants, I would expect that it would also be unhelpful for those who are not depressed. In any event, there is certainly no evidence that the herb benefits people who are not suffering from depression. So it doesn't make sense to go to the expense and trouble of taking St. John's wort and risking potential side effects unless you are feeling depressed.

Is St. John's Wort Useful in the Treatment of Anxiety?

Anxiety is often one of the symptoms of depression, and when it is part of an overall depressed picture, it appears that St. John's wort will help the anxiety along with the other symptoms of depression. Some people, however, suffer from anxiety without exhibiting any symptoms of depression and so far there have been no research studies to determine whether these people will benefit from St. John's wort. It would not be surprising if the herb did prove to be of some value in treating anxiety, since many other antidepressants have been found to be helpful in the treatment of anxiety disorders. As noted earlier in the book, some people with panic disorder, a type of anxiety disorder, have reported improvement in their symptoms after taking St. John's wort. There certainly seems little harm in trying the herbal treatment for a month or two if you are anxious and determining for yourself whether it is helpful to you, but you may want to start with a low dosage and increase it slowly since anxious people may be more susceptible to the symptoms of restlessness reported by some people on St. John's wort.

Can St. John's Wort Help Me Deal with Temporary Stress?

This is an interesting question for which we also have no scientific answers. Nevertheless, several people have told me that they have been helped by the herb when they have used it to deal with the effects of temporary stress and it would be surprising to me if many people are not already using it in this way to good effect. Once again, you might want to try the herb for yourself and see if it helps. I deal with this question more extensively in chapter 2, "St. John's Wort in Everyday Life."

How About Using St. John's Wort for Obsessive-Compulsive Disorder (OCD)?

There are no clinical trial data that address this question. In the treatment of OCD, the most effective drugs are those that selectively target, and are most potent in affecting, the serotonin system. Since St. John's wort has a more balanced action across three different neurotransmitter systems, it might prove to be less effective than the selective serotonin reuptake inhibitors, such as Prozac and Zoloft, in the treatment of OCD. One type of compulsive behavior that is very hard to treat is compulsive hair pulling, also known as trichotillomania. Although there are no studies on the use of St. John's wort for this condition either, I have reported on one serious case in which the patient benefited from the herbal remedy (see chapter 3).

What Can I Do If St. John's Wort Doesn't Work for Me?

Whenever there is an exciting new treatment, it is natural for people to be hopeful that it will be the answer to their problems and disappointed if it is not. Remember that even if St. John's wort is not effective for you by itself, it may still have some value in combination with other antidepressants. Bear in mind, though, that no antidepressant treatment works for everybody, and that must surely be true of St. John's wort as well. Take comfort in the knowledge that there are many other available antidepressants, some old, tried, and tested, some newly arrived, with claims of all kinds of advantages, and others yet to appear on the market. It is very unusual not to be able to find some medication or combination of treatments that will help extricate a person from the murky depths of depression. My approach with my own patients is to keep trying different strategies and, sooner or later, such attempts are almost always successful.

Should I Consider Taking Preparations That Contain Combinations of Different Herbs?

If you look on the shelves of your local health food stores, you will find all sorts of mixtures containing St. John's wort along with other herbal remedies. It has often been mixed with valerian, a mild sleeping medication, and sold as an overall restorative. Such combinations have been marketed in Europe for many years and are available in this country as well. In fact, some of the European studies that have compared St. John's wort with a placebo have used preparations that include valerian. St. John's wort has also been combined with the herbal anti-anxiety compound kava-kava, as well as with any number of other substances, such as passionflower extract. Should you consider taking such preparations, and do they have any advantage over taking St. John's wort alone?

This kind of question does not pertain only to herbal medications, but to synthetic medications as well, where combinations of different medications are made available in a single capsule in an attempt to provide a number of different therapeutic effects. Even though I frequently prescribe combinations of individual medications, in practice I almost never recommend preformulated combinations. The reason for this is very simple. If different medications are doing different things, you need to be able to alter the dosage of each one individually and wait to observe its effects in order to know how best to proceed. A preformulated combination may cause a side effect, for example, and you would not know for sure which of the medications in the formulation was responsible for it. Reasoning along the same lines, I would discourage the use of herbal combinations. Although some of the other herbal remedies may have beneficial effects in their own right, if they are to be tried, I recommend that they be taken individually after you have had a chance to observe the effects of taking St. John's wort by itself. A discussion of the effects of kava-kava and valerian goes beyond the scope of the present book, but they are herbs with valuable therapeutic potential in their own right and I can refer the interested reader to Jean Carper's authoritative and highly readable *Miracle Cures* (HarperCollins, 1997) for a detailed discussion of the herbs and how best to use them.

Be sure to avoid combinations advertised for weight loss, that contain the herb ma huang, also known as ephedra. Ma huang is a potentially dangerous stimulant that has been responsible for several deaths in the United States and is banned in some countries. There is no evidence that St. John's wort is of any benefit in promoting weight loss, though it is conceivable that it may help if the weight gain occurred as part of a depression.

In summary, herbal combinations are not recommended. You may well benefit from taking more than one herb, but each should be taken for a specific purpose, in a particular dosage, and only after you have some knowledge about its potential side effects as well as its potential benefits. In addition, you should add the herbs to the mix one at a time in order to determine what effect each is having.

Is St. John's Wort Addictive?

There is no evidence that St. John's wort is addictive. Though I know of no reports of any withdrawal after St. John's wort is stopped, it is generally better to taper an antidepressant than to stop it abruptly. As with any other antidepressant, however, depressive symptoms may recur when the medication is discontinued.

Can St. John's Wort Work At First and Then Stop Working? What Should I Do If That Happens?

It is not uncommon for an antidepressant that works initially to stop working after a period of time, which may range from weeks to years. This could occur with St. John's wort as well. A relapse of this kind may be due to a worsening of the depression, which is sometimes the result of a definable cause, such as a personal loss, a new stress, or the onset of winter. Wherever possible, the first-line response to such a setback is to deal with the underlying cause, for example, to obtain extra support from friends and family, adopt strategies to help deal with the stress, or increase the amount of environmental light, all of which are described in more detail in earlier chapters.

If the trigger for relapse cannot be identified, or if the steps to correct it by making environmental changes are unsuccessful, medication adjustments can be made, including increasing the dosage of St. John's wort or adding another antidepressant. Sometimes a person develops what is known as a tolerance to an antidepressant, which means that certain chemical changes in the brain override the beneficial effects of the medication. In this case, it can pay to switch to another medication or to add a medication specifically designed to potentiate the effects of the antidepressant. Drugs such as lithium carbonate and synthetic thyroid hormone have been reported to be effective potentiators of conventional antidepressants and may be of value when added to St. John's wort as well. If the medication situation is complicated enough to warrant potentiation of an antidepressant, it is certainly necessary for a highly skilled physician to be involved in treatment decisions. The purpose of providing you with this information is for you to understand some of the steps your doctor is likely to consider in dealing with the delayed development of unresponsiveness to an antidepressant.

One possible reason St. John's wort may stop working is that the composition of active ingredients may vary from one batch of St. John's wort to another. You might suspect this to be the case if you purchased a new batch of St. John's wort just before noticing the change in antidepressant effect. Reliability of quality control is one reason why I recommend the brand of St. John's wort with the best-documented and most reliable track record, namely, Kira, so as to minimize the likelihood of relapses due to inconsistencies between batches.

What Are the Pros and Cons of Using St. John's Wort Versus the SSRIs Such as Prozac and Zoloft?

It is important to remember that there have been no head-to-head trials comparing St. John's wort with the SSRIs in the treatment of depression. All reports of comparisons between the herbal and synthetic antidepressants are therefore anecdotal. Nevertheless, there are lessons to be learned from anecdotes, and one conclusion I have reached, based on many stories such as the ones included in chapter 5, is that there are certain people who do better on St. John's wort than on the SSRIs. When both types of antidepressants are used in their conventional dosages, St. John's wort appears to be superior to the SSRIs with respect to side effects. Particularly, it appears to cause fewer sexual side effects, less weight gain, and fewer feelings of dullness in thinking or feeling. When used in their conventional dosages, it is possible that the SSRIs may be more potent and I have encountered cases in which they have reversed depressive symptoms that did not respond to St. John's wort alone. In the currently planned multicenter research study sponsored by the National Institute of Mental Health, St. John's wort and Zoloft are to be compared for the first time. It will be fascinating to see how they stack up against each other. In the meantime, each depressed person will have to choose the type of antidepressant—herbal or synthetic—best suited to his or her needs based on the information available and personal preferences.

Part III

ST. JOHN'S WORT THROUGH THE AGES

From Ancient Remedy to Herbal Superstar

13

THE HISTORY AND MYTHOLOGY OF ST. JOHN'S WORT

For those who are contemplating taking St. John's wort and are worried about its potential for harmful effects, it will no doubt be a comfort to know that the herb has been recommended for therapeutic purposes for almost two thousand years. But beyond the comfort that comes with history and familiarity, the story of how St. John's wort has emerged from the millions of species that populate the plant kingdom to become a scientifically proven antidepressant is a fascinating one. Over the past two millennia, *Hypericum perforatum* has been singled out for its medicinal properties by eminent medical writers, has been included in the inventories of herbalists and folk healers, and has been the focus of all manner of superstitions. It was only in the last decade, however, that the herb has been subjected to scientific study. In this chapter I will discuss the history and mythology of the herb and will summarize the modern research on St. John's wort in the chapter that follows.

The first person on record who referred to St. John's wort was Pliny the Elder, a Roman born in Como in the first century after the death of Christ. Although he had a prominent military and political career, he is now best known for his writings, including his famous book on natural history. In this work he refers to "hypericon," noting that "the seed is of a bracing quality, checks diarrhoea and promotes urine; it is taken with wine for bladder troubles." A man of enormous intellectual curiosity, Pliny the Elder was ultimately killed by the very trait that was responsible for his great fame. At age fifty-six, he set out to explore the foothills of Mount Vesuvius during the volcano's historic eruption in the first century A.D. and suffocated to death from the fumes.

The next mention of St. John's wort is by Dioscorides, a Roman army surgeon born in Greece. In his medical text, he separated out the different types of hypericum and noted that the fruit of this plant smelled of resin and, when bruised, stained the fingers with liquid resembling blood. He recommended drinking the herb with special liquids, "for it expells many cholerick excrements ... continually until that they be cured," as well as rubbing it on burns. So well regarded was the herb that it is reported to have been an ingredient of a remedy given to the emperor Nero in the first century A.D.

After these two classical authorities, little new was written about St. John's wort for 1,400 years, when a towering medical authority of the Renaissance, Paracelsus, turned his attention to the herb. Paracelsus was his adopted name, a bit grandiose in that it suggested that he transcended the earlier Roman medical authority, Celsus, but more user-friendly than his real name, Philippus Aureolus Theophrastus Bombast of Hohenheim. An iconoclastic man, Paracelsus disparaged much of the formal university teachings of the day, wondering in one of his letters how "the high colleges managed to produce so many high asses." "The universities do not teach all things," he noted, "so a doctor must seek out old wives, gipsies, sorcerers, wandering tribes, old robbers, and such outlaws and take lessons from them. A doctor must be a traveller."

Among his many medical interests and contributions, Paracelsus turned his attention to herbal remedies, which he regarded as an expression of the will of God. He singled out St. John's wort, which he called "The Perforata," as an herb of special importance, occupying a central place in the totality of God's remedies, which he called the "arcanum." He wrote of using St. John's wort to treat three separate conditions: wounds, parasites, and what he called "phantasmata," which appear to be the equivalent of psychotic symptoms, or delusions and hallucinations. But he also recommended St. John's wort for healing the soul. Although he mentioned melancholia in his writings, he did not specifically recommend St. John's wort for this condition.

It was another scientist, about a century later, who in 1630 made the first detailed observations about the value of St. John's wort in the treatment of melancholia. The writer Angelo Sala credited Paracelsus as his major inspiration, but actually, Sala's writings go far beyond those of his predecessor in this regard. Sala is not as famous as some classical authorities, but he was a very impressive man, surprisingly modern in his belief in the use of chemicals to treat illnesses, including those affecting the mind. He observed:

> Saint John's wort has a curious, excellent reputation for the treatment of illnesses of the imagination, which are known by some as phantasmata and by others as mad spirits and for the treatment of melancholia, anxiety and disturbances of understanding, which sometimes affect highly intelligent people whose primary personality is not melancholic and in whom you do not see persistent melancholic humor. Saint John's wort cures these disorders as quick as lightning. It takes a day and a night. With the same power it works against the symptoms caused by witches in a way that is superior—as best I can tell—to the effects of any other type of plant or medication, though these may be very highly respected.

Aside from this being the first clear reference that I can find to the use of St. John's wort as an antidepressant, Sala's comments are of interest for two other reasons. First, he claims an almost immediate antidepressant effect for St. John's wort. This is at odds with the experience of many, who have noted that treatment for at least two to three weeks is needed before an antidepressant effect can be expected. Yet I have certainly encountered individual patients, some of whom are mentioned in the earlier chapters, who have noted an immediate antidepressant effect of the herb. Indeed, if such an immediate effect did not occur at least in some people, it is hard to imagine how the herb would ever have been discovered to have antidepressant properties. Second, it is interesting to note that even though Sala was an enormously gifted clinician, he was nevertheless influenced by the superstitions of the times and apparently believed in the ability of witches to cast their evil spells and in the power of herbs to remove them.

Sala waxes eloquent about the therapeutic effects of the herb:

> In various patients I have found these effects and, without overstating the herb's benefits, I effected cures which you can achieve neither with all the rest of your Apothecary nor with the best prescriptions made out of gold, silver, coral, pearls, stone or jewels (even those that have been found to be useful and wonderful in the treatment of other illnesses). I could not have treated these patients more effectively. I recognize, even as I am describing these cures, that novices who have never had such experiences would be scornful of these claims.

To prepare the hypericum mixture, Sala recommends that the reader chop the petals and leaves (of St. John's wort) and mix them with brandy; put the mixture in a jar and cover it with a large metal cover; put the jar into a warm-water bath; and separate the clear liquid from the sap by decanting it into another glass. He recommends that the prescription be used twice a day, in the morning and evening, for as long as is necessary.

These instructions show that Sala recognized the value of using alcohol to extract the active ingredients of St. John's wort, a process used even to this day in the preparation of hypericum. Putting the mixture in a warm-water bath would make the extraction process more efficient, and placing a metal cover over the mixture would prevent the active ingredients from being broken down by light. Sala's final recommendations, to administer the herbal extract twice a day and to use it as long as is necessary, are in line with modern treatment methods. If one considers that these clinical observations and recommendations were described more than 350 years before the use of Prozac, it is apparent how extraordinary Sala was as a pioneer in the pharmacological treatment of depression.

Before leaving this remarkable man, it is worth considering his attitude toward earlier authorities. He credits them and is highly respectful of their contributions, almost to the point of diminishing his own innovations. But he also emphasizes that it is important to improvise and change the way in which a medication is used in order to make it more potent or effective for a particular condition. In this regard as well, Sala, a little-known seventeenth-century clinician, showed himself to be remarkably modern and open-minded in his attitudes.

For the three centuries after Sala's writings appeared, the use of hypericum for the treatment of melancholia was securely incorporated into the German literature, but was remarkably absent in the British and American literature, which stressed the superficial use of the herb for the treatment of burns and wounds. In the early decades of the present century, scientific interest in hypericum emerged when it became apparent that cattle could develop toxic and sometimes fatal skin reactions after eating large quantities of St. John's wort. Curiously, the skin reactions occurred only on those parts of the hide that were not pigmented and turned out to be caused by the harmful effect of the sun's rays, which broke hypericum into toxic chemicals. Such observations have caused people to question whether toxic reactions of the skin or even the eyes might occur in people who are taking St. John's wort as an antidepressant. The good news is that there is no evidence that St. John's wort, used in therapeutic dosages, is harmful to either the skin or the eyes. It turns out that cattle develop such toxic skin reactions after eating amounts of the herb that are fifty to a hundred times greater than those used therapeutically. Even so, some people do complain of sun sensitivity when on St. John's wort.

The next noteworthy contributor to the history of the antidepressant effects of St. John's wort, a certain Dr. Daniel in Germany, ushered in the modern scientific approach to the herb. Based on experiments with rats, in which he gave the animals hypericum and exposed them to various intensities of light, which produced both agitation and skin problems, Daniel hypothesized that the psychological effects of hypericum might be mediated via the skin. He reported in 1939 that hypericum administered to weakened rats caused them to become more energetic, to eat more, and to gain weight. Influenced by the results of these animal experiments, he began giving hypericum to depressed patients who suffered from loss of appetite and weight, in addition to other depressive symptoms.

Daniel administered liquid extracts of hypericum three times a day for three weeks to sixteen patients with relatively mild depression and observed a favorable response in twelve of the sixteen. This encouraged him to use the extract to treat more seriously depressed patients. He particularly selected depressed patients who had been in a hospital for several years so that he could feel reasonably certain that any observed recovery would be unlikely to occur by chance alone. He undertook his treatment studies before the development of double-blind placebo-controlled studies, which are the current gold standard for good clinical research. In these studies neither the patient nor the treating physician knows whether an active substance or a placebo is being administered. In his studies, Daniel used only the active substance—hypericum extract. Nevertheless, the excellence of his clinical observations and descriptions is quite persuasive. Here is an account of one of Daniel's success stories:

> A 30-year-old male patient, medically and neurologically healthy, had a nervous breakdown five years ago. Three years ago he missed work over a period of three weeks because of an unexpected state of anxiety. Family history is negative. At present the patient believes that he is a bad human being in that he is not able to fulfill his obligations properly. He ruminates during the night

about the following day and is sleeping badly. He tried sleep medications (valerian). In the past two weeks he had no appetite and lost weight. He is crying a lot and has suicidal thoughts.

The diagnosis is reactive depression. The treatment is a vegetarian diet without salt and hydrotherapy, with extract of hypericum, 5 drops three times a day. On the third day of treatment there is a very obvious deterioration of his condition and then he expresses suicidal intentions. The dose is increased to 6 drops three times a day and on the fifth day of this regimen there is a slight improvement in his condition. His dosage is increased further to 7 drops three times a day and on the tenth day of this regimen there is a marked desire to eat and spontaneous sleep. His suppressed self is freed up and 14 days after beginning the treatment he eats enough on a regular basis, sleeps every night for six hours, feels, as the patient himself describes it, "completely changed" and wants to be discharged. This is done after another week when the patient reports being free of all feelings of guilt, strong enough, happy to go to work, and healthy in body and in mind. In addition, there are no objective signs of any depressive symptoms.

Daniel reported eight similar cases with similar responses to hypericum. He observed no relapses in these patients over the course of a year, during which they continued to work and felt fully recovered. Daniel was by no means indiscriminate in his positive reports on hypericum. In contrast to his experience in the treatment of depression, he noted no beneficial effects of hypericum in the treatment of schizophrenia, nor in the type of Parkinsonism that followed the severe flu epidemic (encephalitis lethargica), which was dramatized by Oliver Sacks in his popular book *Awakenings*. Daniel hypothesized that the antidepressant effects of hypericum were mediated via the effects of light absorbed through the skin and acting on circulating hypericum and blood-borne pigments. Nevertheless, he acknowledged that this was all speculative, and emphasized the practical importance of bringing the beneficial effects of hypericum to the reader's attention regardless of the mechanism by which these effects were mediated.

I report the writings of Daniel in detail because in many ways he was surprisingly modern in his approach, moving from animal experiments to human studies, documenting his cases with clarity, testing a hypothesis, and reaching useful conclusions. His case notes are remarkably well written, comprehensive yet succinct. His practice of gradually increasing the dosage of hypericum is right in line with good modern antidepressant treatment, and his dosing regimen—three times a day for three weeks—is identical to that recommended for modern treatment with St. John's wort and employed in many of the modern treatment studies described in the next chapter. One noteworthy point in the above description of the depressed young man is that Daniel persisted with his treatment despite an apparent initial setback, recognizing that a favorable response to antidepressant treatment does not always involve a linear improvement from day one. No doubt the advent of World War II caused Daniel's clinical research—and that of many other German scientists—to lie buried in the history books. It was to take another half a century before hypericum would once again be studied in such a systematic way and, once again, this would occur in Germany.

Fuga Daemonum: The Devil's Scourge

Formerly it was supposed, and not without reason, that madmen were possessed of the devil, and this plant was found so successful in that disorder, that it had the title of Fuga daemonum, as curing demoniacs.

—ROBERT JOHN THORNTON,
A FAMILY HERBAL, 1814

St. John's wort, St. John's wort,
My envy whosoever has thee,

I will pluck thee with my right hand,
I will preserve thee with my left hand,
Whoso findeth thee in the cattlefold,
Shall never be without kine.

—A. CARMICHAEL, *CARMINA GADELICA,* 1900

For centuries St. John's wort has been the focus of innumerable superstitions. It comes into bloom around June 24, St. John's Day, and perhaps for this reason has been named after the saint both in the English-speaking world and in Germany, where it is called *Johanniskraut*. Its spotted petals when rubbed between the fingers yield a red liquid reminiscent of the blood of the martyred saint. With its crown of yellow petals and its delicate yellow raylike filaments, it readily conjures up associations to the sun, which are reinforced by the appearance of its flowers so close to the summer solstice.

In general, St. John's wort has been used to ward off evil spirits, a practice that goes back to the time of the ancient Greeks and Romans. Some consider the very word "hypericon" to be derived from two Greek words, *hyper* (above) and *eikon* (image), indicating its power over apparitions, or spirits. This devil-busting property was formalized in one of the earliest compendiums of drugs, the Salternitan drug list of the thirteenth century, which referred to St. John's wort as *herba demonis fuga,* or the herb that chases away the devil. From that time onward its magical properties were frequently noted and an official medical textbook of the sixteenth century, the *New Kreuterbuch*, referred to St. John's wort as *Fuga demonum,* or the devil's scourge, a term that was repeated frequently in the literature over the next several hundred years. It is tempting to speculate that the antidepressant effects of the herb might have inspired some of these superstitions, given the ignorance about mental illness that abounded over those centuries. If mental illness was the result of demonic possession, surely anything that cured it must be a charm against the devil?

Franciscan monks used the herb in their exorcism rituals in the seventeenth century, and ordinary people would carry the herb around with them. Even Paracelsus and Sala, whose medical writings were so impressive, recommended that people wear the herb in their shirts or under their hats to ward off the spirits that were thought to cause madness. Children wove the herb into garlands and threw them on the roofs of houses to safeguard their inhabitants. The herb was also known as a "love oracle" that could predict the fate of a love affair. Women would press the buds between their fingers, think of their loved ones, and see whether the sap that oozed out of the plant was red or colorless. While doing so, they would chant: "If my lover's good, the blood will run red; if my lover's gone, there'll be only foam." Others would use the plant to determine which member of the family would live the longest. Still others believed that it would repel thunderstorms. Women were instructed to carry the herb on their bodies to keep lusty men at bay, and it was supposed to be especially good for warding off a demon lover. Yet others used it to detect if a witch entered a house (the plant would wilt), or to induce a witch to declare herself. According to one myth, the devil was so angry at the herb's magical powers that he penetrated its leaves with needles, thereby explaining the origin of the perforations. The list of superstitions goes on and on.

These superstitions knew no geographic boundaries and they were rampant throughout Europe and the British Isles. One British account of the magical powers of hypericum appears in John Aubrey's *Miscellanies,* published in 1696.

A House (or Chamber) somewhere in London was Haunted; the Curtains would be rashed at Night, and awake the Gentleman that lay there, who was Musical and a familiar acquaintance of Henry Louis. Henry Louis to be satisfied did lie with him; and the Curtains were rashed so then: The Gentleman grew lean and pale with the frights, One Dr. ___ Cured the House of this disturbance and Mr. Louis said that the principal ingredient was Hypericon put under his Pillow.

Some people will stop at nothing in their quest for scientific truth.

Not everyone went along with these superstitions. Since a number of the herbalists who recommended St. John's wort for its magical properties were women, and many of those in the church and the medical profession, who disapproved of these practices, were men, the skepticism of these men sometimes took on a misogynist edge. This is evident in the title of an early eighteenth-century book on superstitions, *The Philosophy of the Shining Skirts, or The Accurate Investigation of Superstitions Performed by Many Women of Supernatural Brilliance.* A similar tone is struck in the following poem, written by a priest, Conradus Rosbach, at the end of the sixteenth century:

> *Hard Hay is the name of the herb*
> *Usually you find it in very dry places*
> *It's called Johanniskraut or Fuga Demonum*
> *It's superstition and nonsense*
> *Women herbalists who deal extensively in such matters*
> *Should be penalized as soon as possible*
> *So abandon such superstitions*
> *And don't try to save money by avoiding the doctor*

As we arrive at the closing years of the twentieth century, it is as important as ever to separate fact from fancy and science from mythology. Curiously, the question raised by the sixteenth-century priest as to whether one should self-medicate or seek the help of a physician is as relevant today as it was then. I hope that I have answered that question to some degree in this book. When symptoms are mild and there is relatively little at stake, it may be sensible to treat oneself with remedies available without prescription. On the other hand, when symptoms begin to encroach on important areas of one's life or one's physical functioning, such as occurs in cases of major depression or dysthymia, a physician should always be involved.

Although the decision as to whether to self-medicate with

an herbal antidepressant or to seek a physician's help is a personal one, there are also larger political and economic considerations involved when these decisions are made by great numbers of people. These considerations are the subject of the chapter that follows.

14

THE POLITICS AND ECONOMICS OF
ST. JOHN'S WORT

As I have mentioned, in Germany St. John's wort vastly out-sells Prozac, which is the number one–selling prescription drug in the United States. In recent years German doctors have written about seven prescriptions for St. John's wort for every Prozac prescription—and that does not take into account the millions of St. John's wort tablets sold over the counter. There is every reason to believe that St. John's wort can become as popular an antidepressant in this country as it is in Germany, and if that occurs, the sales of the herbal antidepressant will take over a major fraction of the U.S. antidepressant market. The over-the-counter availability of St. John's wort gives the herb the additional market advantage of easier accessibility as compared with prescription antidepressants. Many patients may seek to treat their own depressions as opposed to seeking help from the medical establishment. Whatever the wisdom of such a decision on the part of the patient, this change in behavior will shift money away from doctors and pharmaceutical companies and into the pockets of producers of herbal compounds, owners of health food stores, and, most important, patients themselves.

Insurance companies and health maintenance organizations are in a position to influence the relative cost of St. John's wort versus conventional antidepressants. By choosing to reimburse patients for synthetic antidepressants but not for St. John's wort, which is currently the case in the United States, they can make the herbal antidepressant more expensive than the synthetic ones for some patients. The current situation in

Germany is that St. John's wort is reimbursed if it is prescribed by a doctor but not if it is purchased over the counter. That seems like a reasonable guideline for insurance companies in this country to follow as well.

The questions raised in this chapter, such as "Should people be encouraged to treat their own depressions?" or "Should active antidepressants be available over the counter?," are worth debating in their own right and will no doubt be discussed in the years to come. Given the economic and political stakes involved in these issues, however, it is important for the consumer to be aware of the potential biases of those who are most likely to be engaged in the debate even though it does not invalidate the content of their arguments. With this in mind, let us examine some of the controversies that have been raised in relation to St. John's wort.

Since No U.S. Studies of St. John's Wort Have Been Performed to Date, Should We Reserve Judgment About Its Effectiveness Pending the Conclusion of U.S. Studies?

There does not seem to be much merit in this argument. To my knowledge, there are no antidepressants that have proven to be effective on one side of the Atlantic and not on the other. In the use of St. John's wort to treat depression, the Europeans have been leaders for over 350 years. Since the publication of the findings of Commission E in Germany in the mid-1980s, St. John's wort has been actively studied there. A high-strength preparation of hypericum was developed in Germany, and when tested at a dosage of 900 mg per day it was found to be superior to a placebo in multiple controlled studies. While each of these studies may be flawed or limited in one way or another, taken together they portray a convincing picture of an active antidepressant. While the large U.S. multicenter study currently being undertaken is likely to add valuable new information to our current knowledge, there is already ample evidence from European studies to indicate that St. John's wort is an effective antidepressant. In addition, if we wait several years until the results of the U.S. multicenter study have been ana-lyzed and presented, many depressed people who might stand to benefit from the herbal antidepressant will suffer unneces-sarily while waiting for the results. Many U.S. citizens have already voted with their feet and decided to go ahead and try St. John's wort. I believe they are justified in doing so.

Depression Is a Serious Illness That Should Be Treated by a Doctor

Depression can certainly be extremely serious and, in some cases, even a fatal condition. But the symptoms of depression range in severity from severe to mild instances of feeling stressed and overwhelmed or lacking in energy and enthusi-asm. In this regard, depression is like many medical problems, for example, headaches, which can range from tension headaches to the intense, throbbing pain of migraine or the pressure headaches that may signal the presence of a brain tumor. While tension headaches can be treated simply with painkillers, the more severe headaches need the help of a neu-rologist. Just as you might not consider going to a doctor if you suffered from mild tension headaches, so you might not feel the need to get medical help for mild symptoms of depression or stress.

Regardless of what one believes the ideal course of action in dealing with depression to be, a simple inspection of the num-bers will indicate that it is impossible for all people with depressive symptoms to be taken care of by physicians. According to one estimate, 17.6 million people in the United States suffer from major depression. There are approximately 38,000 psychiatrists and 17,000 general practitioners in this country. If all the depressed people were evenly divided among these providers, that would mean approximately 320 depressed patients for each doctor. Such numbers would pose an over-whelming caseload for a practitioner, who would also be expected to care for patients with other types of disorders as well. In addition, patients with major depression constitute only a fraction of individuals with depressive symptoms. According to one widely respected population study, more than one in five adults complained of depressive symptoms in the month before being surveyed. Many of these were regarded as suffering from what is known as subsyndromal depression, a less marked form of the condition but one nevertheless that is responsible for considerable misery and suffering. Clearly, it is unrealistic to imagine that all of these people could be properly taken care of by the mainstream medical establishment and the evidence bears this out.

In a recent consensus statement in the authoritative *Journal of the American Medical Association*, a group of leading researchers observed:

> *In the Epidemiological Catchment Area study, a nation-wide community survey of psychiatric illness that was conducted around 1980, approximately one third of people suffering from a major depressive disorder sought no treatment for it. Of those who sought treatment, few received adequate treatment. In fact, only about one in ten of those suffering from depression received adequate treatment.*
>
> ROBERT HIRSCHFELD AND COLLEAGUES,
> *JAMA*, 1997

These same authors reviewed the psychiatric histories of people who entered various depression research studies during the years when the SSRIs became very popular, even more recently than 1980, the date of the study cited above, and concluded:

> The lack of any prior antidepressant treatment of patients is striking, ranging from 67% to 48%, who despite being ill for a median of . . . 20 years never received any antidepressant medication. The range of patients who received adequate treatment is also sobering: from a low of 5% to a high of 27%.

Experts in public health have pondered the reasons for people not receiving treatment for their depressive symptoms. In some cases, medical personnel may fail to make the correct diagnosis or treat the problem adequately. In other instances, the depressed person may not recognize the problem, may be embarrassed to seek help for it, may feel afraid of going to a psychiatrist, or may be deterred by the stigma associated with the diagnosis.

Whatever the reasons for the failure of mainstream medicine to adequately take care of depression in a large proportion of affected individuals, there is general agreement that depression is common, exacts a serious toll on the lives of those who suffer from it, and is underdiagnosed and undertreated, and that there is a great deal of room for improvement in the situation.

Where Does St. John's Wort Fit Into the Picture?

John Naisbitt in his best-selling book *Megatrends* observed that one of the major megatrends in recent times is the shift from institutional care to self-care. People want to feel more empowered in terms of taking care of themselves, and this is apparent in all sorts of ways. The U.S. public is becoming increasingly aware of the importance of taking steps to safeguard their own health, such as adhering to certain diets, avoiding tobacco, and wearing seat belts. The public's use of dietary supplements, such as vitamins and minerals, goes well beyond the recommendations of mainstream medicine. According to a recent *New York Times* article, an estimated 100 million Americans are spending approximately 6.5 billion dollars a year on vitamin and mineral supplements, an increase from the 3 billion spent in 1990. The proliferation of self-help groups for addictions, obesity, and specific psychiatric disorders is another example of patients taking their health into their own hands.

The frustration of having to deal with managed care organizations, multiple subspecialists who deal with different parts of the body, high-tech and costly medical procedures, and the depersonalized atmosphere of modern medicine have combined to alienate many patients and keep them from seeking help from doctors. In contrast, the idea of natural treatments, dispensed by a friendly health food store owner and administered by oneself, often seems very appealing, as the story that follows illustrates. St. John's wort has therefore found a ready market in the United States, particularly given the European data in support of its effectiveness and benign side-effect profile. I predict that this trend will continue.

Shirley: Economic Considerations in the Use of St. John's Wort

A fifty-year-old woman writes to me as follows:

> I first heard about St. John's wort as a treatment for depression when I was reading about natural remedies for menopausal symptoms. I began taking 300 mg but did not find that taking one pill was helpful. This past summer my husband suggested I up the dosage to 600 mg and that was the magic amount for the summer. Now that we have switched times [at the onset of autumn], I am taking an additional 300 mg in the afternoon, which helps.
>
> I have been in and out of therapy since I was twenty-five. Therapy with the right therapist(s) is helpful, but it is also expensive and time-consuming. My employer has a cap on the number of hours of therapy a person can undergo, and I am getting closer to that cap every week. I am hoping that this next calendar year is my last year of needing therapy. I was not in therapy for several long periods of my life. Often, a tragedy, such as a death in the family or major surgery, would send me back in.
>
> I prefer natural herbs to drugs wherever I can. I did take Elavil for six months in the '70s. I also took Librax, but had a bad reaction to it. I have refused to take Prozac or Zoloft. I don't think they've been tested long enough, and I really don't want to rely on a drug to control my mood.

Whether or not one agrees with Shirley's opinions about psychotherapy, herbal remedies, or antidepressant medications, she does seem to embody the trend that Naisbitt mentions in his book. I do believe that she speaks for a very large number of people who are concerned about the cost of mental health care, are interested in natural remedies, and are eager to take their health into their own hands as much as possible. St. John's wort provides a solution to all of these concerns. Relatively inexpensive, highly effective, safe, and mild in terms of side effects, it offers millions of people the opportunity to help themselves. It is, of course, critical to know when self-care has reached its limit and when to seek the help of an expert. Shirley appears to be able to make that distinction. It is an important caveat for others to bear in mind as well.

Depression: A Costly Problem and a Profitable Business

A recent study reported the annual cost of depression in the United States to be approximately 43 billion dollars a year. This amount includes the cost of treating the condition and the loss of productivity and positive contribution to the economy resulting from the illness. Even without taking into account the human suffering involved in the condition, depression is considered to be one of the ten costliest medical conditions in the United States.

While depression is costly, its treatment is lucrative. Thus, the antidepressants Prozac and Zoloft are among the best-selling medications in the country, representing billions of dollars of revenue for their manufacturers. Likewise, the treatment of depression is a profitable enterprise for psychiatrists and other mental health providers and for mental health institutions. While these medications, health care providers, and organizations can literally be lifesavers, those who offer these commodities and services have a marked vested interest in maintaining their share of the market. They might be understandably concerned by the advent of an effective, off-prescription alternative treatment for depression. While some concerns about this new way of treating depression are warranted, others may be suspect, motivated by an attempt to protect economic turf.

In all cases, arguments against the self-administration of St. John's wort need to be considered on their merits. For example, a leading psychiatrist was quoted in a recent *Washington Post* article on St. John's wort as saying, "If a drug has enough activity to actually treat something that is real and substantial, then it ought to be administered under somebody's supervision." If you consider the many active drugs available without prescription, which are routinely self-administered to treat real and substantial problems, such as aspirin for arthritis or antihistamines for allergies, it is clear that this argument is not universally applied in other areas of medicine. Nor, in my opinion, does it necessarily apply in psychiatry either. Perhaps the psychiatric establishment has yet to get used to the novelty of an over-the-counter treatment for depression.

In summary, herbal treatments are here to stay, protected by the Dietary Supplement Health and Education Act of 1994. Given the demand for these substances, there is popular support for keeping such herbal extracts and dietary supplements available for general purchase without prescription. The World Health Organization released guidelines in 1992 suggesting how developing countries may incorporate herbal medications into mainstream medicine. According to pharmacologist Jerry Cott of the National Institute of Mental Health, "the essence of these guidelines is that the historical use of a substance is a valid form of safety and efficacy information, in the absence of scientific documentation to the contrary." In 1995, Congress established the NIH Office of Alternative Medicine to indicate its support for alternative medical approaches.

Those who practice mainstream medicine would do well to become acquainted with alternative medical approaches for which reasonable evidence of efficacy exists. Pharmaceutical houses might also profit by embracing the trend and putting their enormous resources toward helping develop these herbal extracts. And, given the effectiveness of these substances and the enormous public interest in them, researchers who study herbal remedies will surely be repaid for their efforts. Ultimately, though, the biggest winners will be those millions of depressed patients who stand to benefit from nature's own pharmacopia. It would be a great shame if politics and economic interests were allowed to stand in the way of their recovery.

APPENDIX

Scale of Well-Being

Please mark with an X on the scale below the way you feel today. Try to pick the same time of day, every day, then carefully review the whole 24 hours and make your decision. Use as the "anchor" points the *best* you have ever felt (on the right) and the *worst* you have ever felt (on the left). Write in the boxes provided what the best and the worst means for you personally. Try not to let the previous day influence you when you score the next new day.

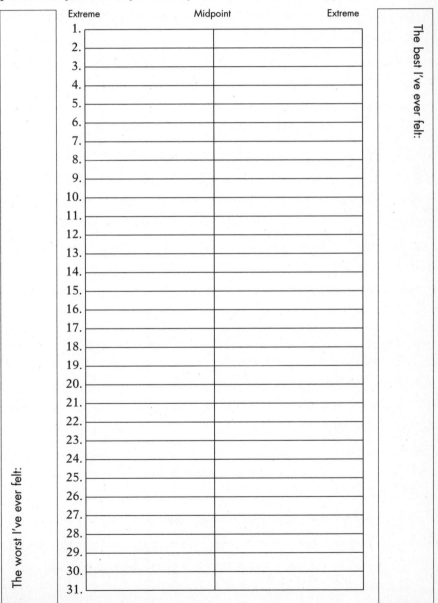

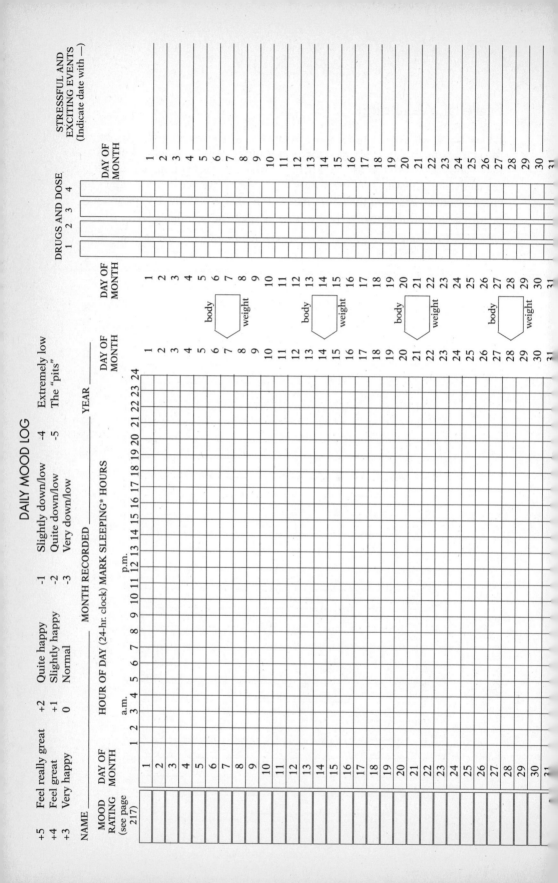

DAILY MOOD LOG

+5 Feel really great	-1 Slightly down/low
+4 Feel great	-2 Quite down/low
+3 Very happy	-3 Very down/low
+2 Quite happy	-4 Extremely low
+1 Slightly happy	-5 The "pits"
0 Normal	

NAME _____

MONTH RECORDED _____ YEAR _____

HOUR OF DAY (24-hr. clock) MARK SLEEPING* HOURS

a.m. 1 2 3 4 5 6 7 8 9 10 11 12 p.m. 13 14 15 16 17 18 19 20 21 22 23 24

MOOD RATING (see page 217)

DAY OF MONTH

DRUGS AND DOSE 1 2 3 4

STRESSFUL AND EXCITING EVENTS (Indicate date with —)

body / weight

SELECTED BIBLIOGRAPHY AND FURTHER READING

Introduction

American Botanical Council, Commission E monographs. (See "Resources.")

St. John's Wort in Everyday Life

Judd, L. L., M. H. Rapaport, M. P. Paulus, and J. L. Brown. "Subsyndromal Symptomatic Depression: A New Mood Disorder?" *Journal of Clinical Psychiatry* 55, suppl. 4 (1994): 18–28.

Liebowitz, M. R., J. M. Gorman, A. J. Fyer, et al. "Social Phobia: Review of a Neglected Anxiety Disorder." *Archives of General Psychiatry* 42 (1985): 729–36.

The Prozac of Herbs

Jacobsen, F. M. "Fluoxetine-Induced Sexual Dysfunction and an Open Trial of Yohimbine." *Journal of Clinical Psychiatry* 53, no. 4 (1992): 199–22.

Ross, J. *Triumph Over Fear*. New York: Bantam Books, 1995.

Science and St. John's Wort: What the Research Shows

Jenike, M. A., ed. *Geriatric Psychiatry and Neurology* 7, suppl. 1 (October 1994): seventeen relevant articles.

Linde, K., G. Ramirez, C. D. Mulrow, A. Pauls, W. Weidenhammer, and D. Melchart. "St. John's Wort for Depression: An Overview and Meta-Analysis of Randomized Clinical Trials." *British Medical Journal* 313 (1996): 253–58.

Müller, W. E., and S. Kasper, eds. *Pharmacopsychiatry* 30, suppl. 2 (September 1997): twelve relevant articles.

Beating the Winter Blues with St. John's Wort and Light

Rosenthal, N. E. *Winter Blues: Seasonal Affective Disorder: What It Is and How to Overcome It.* New York: Guilford Books, 1998.

St. John's Wort in the Elderly

Jenike, M. A., ed. "Editorial," *Journal of Geriatric Psychiatry and Neurology* 7, suppl. 1 (October 1994): S1.

Diagnosing Your Own Depression

Bowlby, J. *Diagnostic Criteria from DSM-IV.* Washington, D.C.: American Psychiatric Association, 1996.

Jamison, K. R. *An Unquiet Mind.* New York: Knopf, 1995.

Making St. John's Wort Part of an Antidepressant Lifestyle

Berger, M., J. Vollmann, F. Hohagen, A. Konig, H. Lohner, U. Voderholzer, and D. Riemann. "Sleep Deprivation Combined with Consecutive Sleep Phase Advance As a Fast-Acting Therapy in Depression: An Open Pilot Trial in Medicated and Unmedicated Patients." *American Journal of Psychiatry* 154, no. 6 (1997): 870–72.

Burns, D. D. *Feeling Good: The New Mood Therapy.* New York: Avon Books, 1992.

Garber, J., and M.E.P. Seligman. *Human Helplessness: Theory and Applications.* New York: Academic Press, 1980.

Frequently Asked Questions About St. John's Wort and a Practical Guide to Its Use

Brown, O. P. *The Complete Herbalist: The People, Their Own Physicians.* 1885.

Burrell, F. A. "Some Uses of the Oleum Hyperici." *New England Medical Monthly* 7 (1887): 342–45.

Carper, J. *Miracle Cures*. New York: HarperCollins, 1997.

Schmidt, U., G. Harrer, U. Kuhn, W. Berger-Deinert, and D. Luther. "Interaction of Hypericum Extract with Alcohol." *Nervenheilkunde* 6 (1993): 314–19.

Sternbach, H. "The Serotonin Syndrome." *American Journal of Psychiatry* 148, no. 6 (1991).

The History and Mythology of St. John's Wort

Aubrey, J. *Miscellanies*. London: Edward Castle, 1696.

Carmichael, A. *Carmina Gadelica*, vol 1. Edinburgh: Norman Macleod, 1900.

Daniel. "Johanniskraut bei psychischen Storungen." *Hippokrates* 10 (1939): 929–32.

Gunther, R. T. *The Greek Herbal of Dioscorides*. New York: Hafner Publishing, 1968.

Guterman, N. *Paracelsus: Collected Writings*. New York: Pantheon Books, 1951.

Jones, W.H.S. *Pliny: Natural History,* vol. 7. Cambridge, Mass.: Harvard University Press, 1956.

Marzell, H. "Johanniskraut eine Volkskundlich: Botanische Studie." *Natur* 10 (1918): 138–40.

Rogers, T. B. "On the Action of St. John's Wort As a Sensitizing Agent for Non-Pigmented Skin." *American Veterinary Review* 46 (1914): 145–62.

Sala, A. *Essentiarum Vegetabilium Anatome*. Rostock, Germany: 1630.

Thornton, R. J. *A Family Herbal*. 2d ed. London: Crosby, 1814.

Vickery, A. R. "Traditional Uses and Folklore of Hypericum in the British Isles." *Economic Botany* 35 (1981): 289–95.

The Politics and Economics of St. John's Wort

Brody, J. E. "In Vitamin Mania, Millions Take a Gamble on Health." *New York Times,* October 26, 1997: A1.

Cott, J. M. "In Vitro Receptor Binding and Enzyme Inhibition By Hypericum Perforatum Extract." *Pharmacopsychiatry* 30, suppl. 2 (1997): 108–11.

Hirschfeld, R., et al. "The National Depressive and Manic-

Depressive Association Consensus Statement on the Undertreatment of Depression." *JAMA* 277, no. 4, (1997): 333–40.

Naisbitt, J. *Megatrends*. New York: Warner Books, 1988.

Okie, S. "Herbal Relief." *Washington Post*, Health section, October 14, 1997: 12.

Regier, D. A., et al. "The De Facto U.S. Mental and Addictive Disorders Service System: Epidemiologic Catchment Area Prospective 1-Year Prevalence Rates of Disorders and Services." *Archives of General Psychiatry* 50 (1993): 85–94.

Santiago, J. M. "The Costs of Treating Depression." *Journal of Clinical Psychiatry* 52, no. 11 (1993): 425–26.

RESOURCES

Author's Web site: http://www.normanrosenthal.com

Further Information About Herbal Medicines

American Botanical Council
P.O. Box 201660
Austin, TX 78720
Fax: 512-351-1924
E-mail: custserv@herbalgram.org
http://www.herbalgram.org

Carper, Jean. *Miracle Cures*. New York: HarperCollins, 1997.

Volker, Schulz, Hänsel Rudolf, and E. Tyler Varro. *Rational Phytotherapy*. New York, Springer, 1998.

Support Groups Geared Specifically to the Treatment of Depression

National Depressive and Manic Depressive Association
    (NDMDA)
730 N. Franklin, #501
Chicago, IL 60610
Tel: 800-826-3632
http://www.ndmda.org

Depression and Related Affective Disorders Association
    (DRADA)
Johns Hopkins University School of Medicine
Meyer 3-181
600 N. Wolfe St.
Baltimore, MD 21287-7381
Tel: 410-955-4647
http://www.med.jhu.edu/drada

National Foundation for Depressive Illness
P.O. Box 2257
New York, NY 10116
Tel: 800-239-1295

Office of Scientific Information
National Institute of Mental Health
5600 Fishers Lane, Room 7C02 MSC 8030
Bethesda, MD 20892
Tel: 800-421-4211
http://www.nimh.nih.gov

INDEX

Abandonment, 21–24
Abdominal discomfort, 49–50, 81,
    117, 172, 178
ADD, *see* Attention deficit disorder
    (ADD)
Addictions:
    recovery groups for, 146–48, 211
    St. John's wort as nonaddictive,
    190
Addison's disease, 48
Adele (case study), 6–8
Adolescents, depression in, 169, 170
Adrenal glands, 98
    tumors of, 129–30
"Advice to Melancholics," 135
Agoraphobia, 28–29
Alcohol, 15, 160
    combined with St. John's wort,
    185
    depression related to use of, 105,
    131, 137, 150, 185
    driving and, 150
    to extract active ingredients of St.
    John's wort, 165, 198
    watching intake of, 149–50, 185
Alcoholics Anonymous, 147
Alice in Wonderland, 64
Alternative medicine, 33
American Botanical Council, 223
American Psychiatric Association,
    103
Amitriptyline, 78
Anhedonia, 84, 85, 92–94, 104, 159
Animals, stress response of, 100, 143
Anna (case study), 78–80
Anorexia, 42
Antibiotics, 37
Antidepressants:
    abruptly discontinuing, 181
    bipolar disorder and, 177
    combined with St. John's wort,
    60–63, 122–26, 170, 181–85, 191
    conditions other than depression
    and, 25–26, 28
    half-life of, 181–82

meta-analysis studies, 32–35
during pregnancy, 170–71
profitability for drug companies,
    213
switching to St. John's wort from,
    52–53, 122–26, 180–82
withdrawal symptoms, 181–82
see also specific drugs
Antiviral agents, 43–44
Anxiety, 7–8, 42, 187
    as side effect, 179
Appetite, 98, 99–100, 104, 106
Atropine, xv
Attention deficit disorder (ADD),
    63–64, 65, 130–31, 133
Aubrey, John, 204
Awakenings (Sacks), 201

Beck, Dr. Aaron, 156
Bed-wetting, 43
Bereavement, 11, 142
Berger, Dr. Mathias, 153
Binge eating, 25
Biological disturbances,
    depression and, 98–101,
    104, 106
Bipolar disorder, 111, 176–78
Blood pressure, 40
Blues, 12–13
Bowel, 40
Bowlby, John, 100
Brands of St. John's wort, 7, 29,
    116–17, 166–68, 190–91
Brandy to extract active ingredients
    of St. John's wort, 165, 198
Brent (case study), 59
British Medical Journal,
    32, 33, 36
Brockmöller, Dr. Jürgen, 37
Brown, Dr. O. Phelps, 164–65
Bulimia, 28, 42, 43
Bupropion, 39
Burns, David, 159
Burrell, F. A., 163
Caffeine, 15

225

Fisch, Dr. Joachim, 153–54
Flight into health, 143–45
Folk healers, 43
"Fortune-telling," 158
Foxglove, xv
Franciscans, exorcisms by, 203
Frankl, Victor, 93
Fred (case study), 63
Freelancing, 143–44
Frieda (case study), 83–85
Friends as social support, 145–46,
191
Frightening thoughts, dealing with,
156–59
Fun, lacking capacity to have,
92–94, 104
Future, gloomy view of the, 101

Gabrielle (case study), 82–83
Gaia, 180
Galileo, 3
Gambling, compulsive, 160
Game plan for use of St. John's
wort, 113–26
currently not being treated for
depression, 114–22
major depressive disorder or
dysthymia, 119–22
mildly blue, stressed-out
category, 115–19
severity of depression,
determining, 114–15
currently on one or more
antidepressants or mood-
regulating drugs, 122–26
doing well and, 124
not doing as well as would
like to, 124–26
questions to ask before first time
use, 113–14
summary, 126
Gerda (case study), 81
German Federal Health Agency,
xv–xvi, 31
Germany, xiii–xiv, xvi, 31, 80–82,164,
178, 199, 200–202, 203, 207, 208
Greta (case study), 77–78, 79
Grieving, 11
Guilt, feelings of excessive, 105

Hair pulling, compulsive, 26–28, 43,
188

Half-life of drugs, 181–82
Hamilton Depression Rating Scale,
78
Health food stores, 207
Health maintenance organizations,
207–208, 211
Healthy pleasures, cultivating,
159–60
Heart problems, 81
Henry (case study), 53–56
Herbal remedies:
companies producing, 207
legislative protection for, 214
resources, 223
St. John's wort combined with
other, 33, 189–90
WHO guidelines, 214
see also specific herbal remedies
Herb Pharm, 180
Herpes, 44
Hippius, Hanns, 166
Hirschfeld, Robert, 210
History and mythology of St. John's
wort, 195–206
HIV, 44
Hopelessness, 106
Hyperforin, 44, 166
Hypericin, 44, 166
Hypericum perforatum, see St. John's
wort (*Hypericum perforatum*)
Hypomanic episodes, 111, 125, 174,
177–78, 179
Hypothalamus, 98
Hysteroid dysphoria, 144–45

Illness in a loved one, 12
Imipramine, 35, 43
Indigestion, 58, 117, 172
Insomnia, 13–15, 98–99, 106
Insurance companies, 207–208
Internet, 9
Interpersonal skills and stress,
139–42
Irene (case study), 81
Irritability, 179

Jake (case study), 57–59
James (case study), 49–50
Jamison, Dr. Kay Redfield, 96–97
Jarsin brand, 167–68
Jenike, Dr. Michael, 75, 76
Jet lag, 137